Alternative Treatments
for
Arthritis

AN *A to Z* Guide

By Dorothy Foltz-Gray

APR

Alternative Treatments *for* Arthritis

AN *A* to *Z* Guide

By Dorothy Foltz-Gray

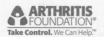

ARTHRITIS
FOUNDATION®
Take Control. We Can Help.™

An Official Publication of the Arthritis Foundation

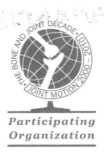

Participating
Organization

Alternative Treatments for Arthritis: An A to Z Guide

By Dorothy Foltz-Gray

An Official Publication of the Arthritis Foundation

Copyright 2005
Arthritis Foundation
1330 West Peachtree Street
Suite 100
Atlanta, GA 30309

Library of Congress Card Catalog Number: 2005921874

ISBN: 0-912423-47-1

Printed in the United States of America

This book was conceived, designed and produced by the Arthritis Foundation. The mission of the Arthritis Foundation is to improve lives through leadership in the prevention, control and cure of arthritis and related diseases.

Editorial Director: SUSAN BERNSTEIN
Art Director and Cover Designer: TRACIE BULLIS
Production Artist: JILL DIBLE

APR 07

Contents

Contents *continued*

The A to Z Listing of
Alternative Treatments

Acknowledgments

Alternative Treatments for Arthritis: An A to Z Guide was written to help those with any form of arthritis, as well as their families and loved ones. The book is the culmination of efforts by physicians, healthcare professionals, Arthritis Foundation volunteers and staff, writers, editors, and designers. The editorial director of the book is Susan Bernstein. The art director and cover designer is Tracie Bullis, and the layout was done by Jill Dible.

We extend thanks to the author, Dorothy Foltz-Gray, a contributing editor of *Arthritis Today,* Arthritis Foundation's monthly magazine and the editor of *The Guide to Good Living with Fibromyalgia* (Arthritis Foundation, 1999). She is also a contributing editor of *Health* and *Alternative Medicine* magazines. James McKoy, MD; Marilyn Barrett, PhD; and Michele Boutaugh, RN, reviewed the book for accuracy.

Ths book is not meant to provide advice or suggestions for your personal medical treatment. Please consult your physician before trying any alternative treatment, or to answer any questions you may have.

*I*ntroduction

Approximately 66 million Americans have some form of arthritis, one of the most widespread conditions in the United States. There are one hundred or more varieties of the disease, all of them painful, resulting in stiff or swollen joints. The most common forms are osteoarthritis, affecting 21 million Americans, and rheumatoid arthritis, affecting 2.1 million, or one percent of American adults. Arthritis is the leading cause of disability in the United States.

The prevalence of arthritis doesn't make it any easier to bear. Not only do some forms – like fibromyalgia and rheumatoid arthritis – take time to diagnose but effective treatment can be frustratingly elusive. Most people start out following medical regimens prescribed by rheumatologists, physicians who specialize in the treatment of arthritis. Patients may try a combination of prescription anti-inflammatories or disease-modifying drugs; over-the-counter pain relievers like acetaminophen; antidepressants, muscle relaxants, or topical treatments like anti-inflammatory gels. They may try steroid injections or surgery. And in almost all cases, their doctors advise exercise and maintaining a healthy weight.

Despite the range of traditional medical options, the same treatments don't work on everyone, and finding a successful regimen sometimes requires trial and error. Increasingly, arthritis patients are considering complementary and alternative treatments, or CAM, which can include anything from herbs to massage to yoga. In fact, according to the National Center for Complementary and Alternative Medicine

(NCCAM) of the National Institutes of Health, 36 percent of American adults use some form of CAM; that figure jumps to 62 percent if megavitamin therapy and prayer are included. And as more and more studies reveal positive results with a number of the treatments, traditional medical practitioners are more comfortable with such choices, and may even suggest them as an adjunct to traditional remedies.

Some of the therapies, like massage, may involve manipulation of sore muscles and joints. Others, like meditation or relaxation techniques, address the psyche: theoretically, by lowering stress levels, sore muscles relax, lowering pain. And some, like yoga, relieve pain through movement, decreasing stiffness and increasing flexibility.

Clearly, if you are reading this book, you probably already have an interest in alternative medicine – or at least the hope that it might help you. Within these pages, you'll find a storehouse of information that can help introduce you to therapies that you can discuss with your doctor. The Arthritis Foundation offers this springboard to reputable information in part because simply scrolling the Internet for information about CAM can be both confusing and overwhelming. Knowing what sites and information are reliable can be a tough call. That's why we've done at least some of that work for you. But whatever you do, don't try any of these methods without consulting your doctor first. Various herbal preparations, for example, can interact with medications you are already taking. Together, you and your physician can assess what's best for you.

The Arthritis Foundation is committed to helping all those with arthritis. In addition to this book, it offers a range of books, brochures and videos, and its monthly magazine, *Arthritis Today*, which reports on the latest in treatments and research. Our Web site, www.arthritis.org, also presents up-to-date news about treatments and research, and message boards on which you can discuss issues with others who have arthritis. It also lists arthritis-related events such as the Arthritis Walk, and programs, community activities and free educational materials.

The Arthritis Foundation also has chapters and branch offices nationwide that offer programs for those with arthritis, including self-help and exercise classes. The foundation also raises money every year for medical researchers working on treatments and knowledge that may one day lead to cures for arthritis and related diseases. For more information, contact your local chapter. You can find your nearest office by calling (800) 568-4045 or by visiting the Arthritis Foundation website, www.arthritis.org. You may also purchase books and videos on our website, or by calling (800) 283-7800.

Chapter I
Understanding Alternative Treatments

WHAT IS AN ALTERNATIVE TREATMENT?

Many alternative treatments are the mainstream medicine of the past – herbal remedies, for example, practiced before the technical advances of the last half century or so. And many, like meditation, have been followed for centuries, and still are considered mainstream medicine in other cultures. But Western notions of mainstream medicine have shifted with medical progress. According to the NCCAM, alternative treatments are those that fall outside the practice of conventional medicine advanced by medical doctors (MDs) or doctors of osteopathy (DOs) and related professionals such as psychologists, physical therapists and registered nurses.

The range of alternative treatments is broad – from herbs to massage to mind-body practices. Below is a quick primer of just what they include:

HERBS, SUPPLEMENTS, AND VITAMINS

Available in health food and grocery stores without a prescription, these are sold without rigorous testing by the U.S. Food and Drug Administration (FDA), and many don't have scientific studies to back their claims. Herbs can come fresh, freeze-dried, or as extracts formed into capsules or tablets. Extracts are also used to make tinctures, usually with an alcohol base. Infusions are liquids made from soaking the herbs in hot water for ten to 15 minutes. Supplements can include vitamins, minerals, amino acids, enzymes, herbs or other plants in capsules or tablets – and they are considered foods, not drugs. But just like drugs, to work they affect your body. Sometimes, just like a drug, they may cause harm. And some may interact negatively with drugs you already take. Always check with your doctor before taking any supplement or herb.

BODYWORK AND MANIPULATIVE THERAPIES

There are more than one hundred types of bodywork, hands-on therapies that involve manipulation or touching of the body. These range from Swedish massage, a full-body kneading of the top layer of muscles, to Asian methods that apply finger and hand pressure on specific points to release energy flow, or qi (pronounced chee). Some methods – like reiki and therapeutic touch – don't actually use touch at all, focusing instead on guiding spiritual energy. The various therapies can help stretch tight muscles, improve flexibility, relieve pain, and help relieve stress and depression that often accompany arthritis.

MIND-BODY/MEDITATIVE TREATMENTS

Although Western medicine has tended to focus on physical symptoms, doctors and researchers are increasingly recognizing the mind's influence on the body. Stress, for example, ups the risk of high blood pressure and heart disease, and lowers immune system defenses. Stress can also augment pain and depression. Mind-body treatments like meditation and relaxation exercises work by lowering stress, which in turn calms body systems, lowering heart and breathing rate and blood pressure.

Some of these techniques like meditation have been practiced since ancient times. Others like cognitive-behavior therapy began as recently as the 1960s. No one treatment is for everyone, and the choices are plentiful including biofeedback, meditation, visualization and guided imagery, hypnosis, relaxation exercises, stress reduction and relaxation programs.

ALTERNATIVE EXERCISE APPROACHES

Exercise is not just for fun anymore. Study after study indicates that exercise can help relieve the pain and stiffness of arthritis as well as lift spirits. Alternative forms of exercise originating from the Far East like yoga, tai chi and qi gong help strengthen muscles and improve blood flow to aching joints and muscles, and release feel-good endorphins without the strain of more traditional exercises. More modern forms of exercise like the Alexander technique, Feldenkrais method and Trager approach are designed to help you move more easily – and for those with arthritis that may mean learning to move in ways that minimize pain.

ALTERNATIVE HEALTH APPROACHES/PHILOSOPHIES

The approaches that Westerners consider "alternative" are in fact mainstream medicine for much of the world. According to the National Center for Complementary and Alternative Medicine, only 10 to 30 percent of medicine practiced worldwide is traditional medicine. The other major healing systems include Ayurveda, the 5,000-year-old healing tradition of India. Its principles emphasize the balance of energy within body and soul. Treatment is non-invasive and includes recommendations similar to the practical advice of Western practitioners – a low-fat diet full of fruits and vegetables, plenty of exercise and rest.

Chinese medicine is another ancient system – 2,000 years old – that focuses on balance between energies. Its most commonly known forms in the West are acupuncture and herbal medicine. Its principles center around the notion of "qi" (pronounced chee), considered the life energy that flows through the body in channels called meridians. Blocked or out-of-balance qi leads to illness.

Naturopathy stems from European practices of the 19th century that focus on prevention and the body's ability to heal itself. Treatments include changes in diet and exercise, the use of herbs and dietary supplements, homeopathy, spinal manipulations, hydrotherapy and counseling. Naturopathic physicians, or NDs, graduate from a four-year training program.

Homeopathy has a long history in Europe and was widely practiced in the United States until the 1950s. The theory behind it is that "like cures like." In other words, giving people a diluted form of what causes the illness will be its cure. Like Ayurveda and Chinese medicine, homeopathy focuses on life force or energy. Remedies are often in the form of tinctures, tablets or creams.

ALTERNATIVE TREATMENTS AND ARTHRITIS: WHY PEOPLE WITH ARTHRITIS SEEK ALTERNATIVE THERAPY

People with arthritis seek alternative treatments for a number of reasons. Some people grow frustrated by relentless pain without a cure, and they are willing to try anything to improve their lot. For others, alternative remedies offer a greater sense of control over the disease than conventional medicine alone. By trying out various practices like massage or yoga, they feel more active in their care. For still others, alternative medicine complements conventional treatments providing relief from stress, depression, pain or stiffness. Some like the personal touch and less hurried visits alternative practitioners often provide. Still, alternative medicine holds no cure for arthritis. Used wisely and in partnership with your doctor, however, these remedies may make you feel better mentally and physically.

Chapter **II**

What You Should Know About Alternative Treatments

THE CONTROVERSY OF USING ALTERNATIVES

Many alternative therapies do not have FDA approval or the backing of rigorous scientific research. And unfortunately a lot of misinformation and faulty claims clog the Internet. So it's essential to consult with your doctor and do some research before using any new therapy, making sure that the information you gather comes from a trusted source. (See *How to Be a Savvy Patient/Consumer,* p. 18.) Before you use any treatment, understand the therapy's possible risks and benefits. And investigate how a new treatment will affect your particular condition and the medications you are already taking. Some therapies have been used safely for hundreds of years; newer treatments have less research or history to back them. It's especially important to be well informed about herbs and supplements. They are "natural" but they are also drugs that can be dangerous if misused, or interact with drugs you already take. Alternative medicines are also controversial simply because they lie outside the mainstream of Western medicine; many doctors are uncomfortable recommending them due to lack of knowledge about them or lack of scientific research.

THE COMPLEMENTARY APPROACH

Alternative therapies are often used in conjunction with conventional treatments to complement the treatments you are already using. This practice is called complementary medicine. For example, you may be taking medication for swollen, inflamed joints but your doctor may also recommend massage therapy or hydrotherapy as a helpful accompaniment to his prescriptions. According to studies at Harvard Medical School, most people use alternative therapies not to replace conventional treatments but to augment their conventional care. And as more and more research backs these treatments, conventional doctors are becoming increasingly comfortable with integrating such practices into their own treatment programs.

TALKING TO YOUR DOCTOR ABOUT ALTERNATIVES

If you do plan on using alternative medicine, the most important first step is to discuss your plans with your doctor. Take this book and any other research you uncover with you when you meet with your doctor. Let him help you explore what you can expect from an alternative treatment in benefits, risks, costs and interaction with traditional treatment. Talk about what signs of improvement to look for and how long you should give a treatment to work. Some doctors, however, are uncomfortable with remedies that fall outside conventional medical training – although this is beginning to change as more research is done on alternative methods. If your doctor disapproves, you can try speaking to another doctor, or even changing to a doctor more comfortable with an integrated approach. But regardless of how your doctor feels about alternative medicine, for your own protection, keep him informed of any treatments you plan to try.

WHY ALTERNATIVES CAN BE POWERFUL: INTERACTIONS, SIDE EFFECTS AND CAUTIONS

Some alternative therapies recommend things like fasting or a restricted diet. Others recommend herbs and supplements. Any measure that drastically changes what you eat can put stress on your body, especially one already taxed by illness. And although herbs and supplements may be "natural" products, nonetheless they are essentially drugs unregulated by the FDA (except for homeopathic remedies and vitamins). Just like synthetic medicines, they can have powerful effects – including unwanted side effects – and can interact with drugs you are already taking. The fact that they are unregulated also means that the preparations aren't standardized. One brand of St. John's wort, for example, may differ from another brand's version. Nor do the bottles have to contain what the labels say they do. In fact, when an independent lab (ConsumerLab.com, 2004) tested sixteen brands of St. John's wort, only ten passed the review. One had less than one quarter of the recommended dose of St. John's wort; three contained levels of metal (cadmium) higher than acceptable by the World Health Organization, and two did not identify what part of the herb they used. Labels may not, however, claim to treat, cure or prevent a disease; otherwise they are considered a drug and their sale illegal. That's why supplements often carry a disclaimer. The American Society of Anesthesiologists suggests patients stop taking herbal supplements two to three weeks before any surgery.

POSSIBLE NEGATIVE EFFECTS OF ALTERNATIVES (HISTORICAL CASES, POSSIBLE INTERACTIONS)

Many herbs and supplements are harmless. But some have the potential to harm. For example, St. John's wort can interfere with iron absorption and birth control pills, increase sunburn risk, and increase the effects of alcohol, sedatives and tranquilizers. Ginger and ginkgo can interfere with warfarin (*Coumadin*, a blood thinner) and aspirin. Ginkgo and other herbs can also increase risk of excessive bleeding. The herbs comfrey and kava kava have been linked to liver damage. Kava kava has also been linked to four deaths. Great Britain and other European countries have banned its sale, and in 2002 FDA issued a warning about its use – as it did about comfrey in 2001. In February 2003 the FDA banned the sale of the popular diet supplement ephedra, or ma huang, because of its link to heart attacks, strokes and death.

Interactions of Supplements with Drugs

Herbs and supplements have their own drug-like powers. When they are combined with prescription or over-the-counter drugs, they may cause unwanted and sometimes dangerous, even fatal interactions. Below are interactions to be aware of:

• **Bromelain** – May augment effects of blood-thinning drugs and tetracycline antibiotics.

• **Capsaicin (or capsicum)** – Increases the absorption and effect of ACE inhibitors (medications used for diabetic kidney disease, heart failure, high blood pressure); some asthma medications, sedatives and antidepressants.

• **Chondroitin** – May augment effects of blood-thinning drugs and herbs.

• **Comfrey** – May affect liver function or cause liver damage or death.

• **Echinacea** – May interfere with immune-suppressant drugs such as corticosteroids taken for lupus and rheumatoid arthritis. May increase side effects of methotrexate.

• **Evening Primrose Oil** – May neutralize effects of anti-convulsant drugs.

• **Fish oil** – May increase effects of blood-thinning drugs and herbs.

• **G.L.A.** – May augment effects of blood-thinning drugs and herbs.

- **Garlic** – May augment effects of blood-thinning drugs and herbs. May decrease the effect of immunosuppressants.

- **Ginger** – May augment the side effects of NSAIDs and effects of blood-thinning drugs and herbs. May also lower blood pressure and blood sugar levels.

- **Ginkgo** – May augment effects of blood thinning drugs, antidepressants and herbs. Also affects insulin levels.

- **Ginseng** – May augment effects of blood-thinning drugs, estrogens and corticosteroids and interact with MAO inhibitors. May also lower blood sugar levels.

- **Kava Kava** – May augment effects of alcohol, sedatives and tranquilizers. Has also been linked to liver damage and failure.

- **Magnesium** – May interact with blood pressure medications.

- **Sarsaparilla** – May increase the absorption of digitalis (an ingredient in some heart medications) and bismuth (an ingredient in some diarrhea medications).

- **St. John's wort** – May increase effects of narcotics, alcohol and antidepressants; increase sunburn risk; interfere with the absorption of iron and with birth control pills, drugs for HIV/AIDS and cancer.

- **Valerian** – May boost effects of sedatives and tranquilizers.

- **Zinc** – May interfere with corticosteroids and other immunosuppressants.

How to Be a Savvy Patient/Consumer

You can increase the chances that your choices of alternative therapies are sound by doing research on your own before diving into any therapy. What are the risks and benefits a therapy offers, particularly to someone who has your form of arthritis? What studies and research support the therapy's claims? If you're investigating a product, look it up on the manufacturer's website to see what studies from scientific journals are listed. Check out independent sites as well. But don't believe everything you see on a website or hear in an advertisement. Ask your doctor and pharmacist for advice. Even if they are not familiar with the therapy, they can probably refer you to a knowledgeable professional.

WHERE TO FIND INFORMATION ABOUT ALTERNATIVES

The Internet is a great place to start searching for data on alternatives but make sure you're surfing reliable sites. One place to start is CAM on PubMed, www.nlm.nih.gov/nccam/camonpubmed.html. The site, developed by the National Center for Complementary and Alternative Medicine and the National Library of Medicine, offers peer-reviewed articles (meaning people in the same field have verified each article's accuracy). Another database, the International Bibliography Information on Dietary Supplements (IBIDS), is not quite as easy to use and can involve waits but the information is reliable. Its address: http://ods.od. nih.gov/databases/ibids. html. You can also check out the FDA's web site, which includes a Center for Food Safety and Applied Nutrition section on dietary supplements (www.cfsan.fda.gov). You can find product recalls and safety alerts at www.fda.gov/opacom/7alerts.html and at the Federal Trade Commission's Diet, Health and Fitness Consumer Information site, www.ftc.gov/bcp/menu-health.htm.

Several other databases also provide information about herbs and supplements: The Natural Medicines Comprehensive Database (www.naturaldatabase.com) lists information about more than 1,000 herbs and supplements, including studies. A subscription costs $92 per year. Another, Natural Standard (www.naturalstandard.com), has solid, peer-reviewed information about all alternative treatments including herbs and supplements. An annual subscription cost $99.

When you check out other sites, NCCAM suggests you evaluate them using these questions:

- Who runs the site? That information should be on every page.

- Who pays for the site? Advertisers? A supplement manufacturer?

- What is the site's purpose? (Click on "About this site.")

- Where does the information come from? Sources should be listed.

- How is the information selected and reviewed? Is there an editorial advisory board?

- How current is the information? Materials should be dated.

- How does the site choose links to other sites? Some require link standards; others accept paid links without review.

- How much information does the site ask you to provide? Some ask you to become a member. If so, check the privacy policy. And make sure the site is secure before offering any personal or financial information.

- How does the site handle interactions with visitors? Is there a way to contact the site's owner. Are chat rooms or forums moderated?

After you've done the research, evaluate the evidence. Choose another therapy if you cannot find any reputable studies about it and the only "evidence" comes from customers. And, of course, dismiss anything that claims to work by secret formula or that touts itself as a cure. And avoid any practitioner who asks you not to see a medical doctor.

To protect yourself when you actually pick out a product, look for the USP (United States Pharmacopeia) on the label, which indicates that it meets the USP standard for strength, purity, packaging and labels and for FDA- or USP-accepted use. Another mark, NF (National Formulary) indicates the supplement meets the USP standard but not the FDA or USP accepted use. But neither mark means the supplement is effective.

To find an alternative practitioner, again, start with your doctor. Or you can also contact a hospital or medical school for referrals. You can also check with the professional organization or state licensing board for the therapy you are considering. Once you have some names, ask for an initial meeting. Ask about training and qualification, experience in working with someone who has arthritis, how effective the therapy may be for arthritis, and anyrelated research available about the procedure. Ask too how many patients he sees per day and for how long, how much he charges and whether it is covered by insurance. Ask what happens during an initial visit and subsequent visits, and how many visits you can expect to have. Ask how his treatments work with the conventional treatments you already receive and how he will work with your doctor. Finally, leave the visit with his brochure and website address.

PAYING FOR ALTERNATIVES: INSURANCE COVERAGE ISSUES

Few alternative treatments are covered by insurance, although that is changing. According to a 2002 survey by America's Health Insurance Plans, 87.4 percent of insurance companies cover at least one type of alternative treatment. Several states – Arkansas, Illinois, Indiana, Nevada, South Dakota, Utah and Wyoming – require insurance companies to cover treatments by any licensed health professional. Washington requires coverage for acupuncture, chiropractic, massage therapy, and naturopathy. You may boost your chances of coverage by asking your doctor to refer you to an alternative practitioner or to "prescribe" supplements since insurance companies are more likely to consider coverage if your doctor deems treatments medically necessary. Chiropractic, acupuncture and massage therapy may be covered but herbs and supplements likely are not. And it's a good idea to let your insurance company know what alternative treatments you would like covered and to ask what its plan offers.

Chapter III
What Is Arthritis?

Arthritis comes in more than one hundred forms but most are characterized by pain, inflammation and stiffness in the joints, the spot where your bones meet, such as your knee or hip. The bone ends lie in a capsule and are covered in cartilage, which helps absorb shock and keeps the bones from rubbing together. Synovial tissue lines the joints, secreting fluid that helps them move. Muscles and tendons also help them move and add support. Different kinds of arthritis affect joints in different ways, even changing their shape and alignment. Some forms of arthritis also affect skin and organs.

Unfortunately, little is known about causes for arthritis. Some, like rheumatoid and psoriatic arthritis, are autoimmune diseases, meaning the immune system attacks itself by mistake. Osteoarthritis may be triggered by injury. In some forms of arthritis, genetics play a role.

COMMON TYPES OF ARTHRITIS

Osteoarthritis: The most common form of arthritis, osteoarthritis affects 21 million Americans, most of whom are over age 45. Also called degenerative joint disease, it involves the breakdown of joint cartilage, causing the bones – particularly weight-bearing bones like knees and hips – to rub together, which in turn brings on pain and immobility. Osteoarthritis has several causes: obesity, which adds wear to the joints, particularly the knees; joint injuries from sports, work activity, or accidents; and genetics. A person can be born with defective cartilage, which may over time cause cartilage breakdown and inflammation. Treatments include pain relievers, exercise, application of cold or heat, and possibly surgery to replace damaged joint components.

Rheumatoid arthritis: RA results from an abnormality of the body's immune system causing inflammation, which begins in the joint lining, and can damage both cartilage and bone. Approximately 2.1 million people in the United States suffer from rheumatoid arthritis – almost 75 percent of whom are women. Most often it begins in middle age, but it can begin as early as age 20. Juvenile arthritis even occurs in children as young as 2. Treatments can include drugs, exercise, hot or cold compresses, and possibly surgery.

Fibromyalgia: Unlike other forms of arthritis, fibromyalgia does not damage joints or cause inflammation. Instead it generates widespread pain in the muscles, tendons and ligaments, accompanied by debilitating fatigue. The condition is characterized by 11 to 18 tender points – points that are sensitive to pressure – located in all areas of the body. As many as 3.7 million Americans have the condition, women more than men. Its cause is unclear, although researchers suspect emotional or physical stress may be involved. Treatments may include exercise, sleep therapy and medication.

Osteoporosis: As people age, most lose bone faster than they can replace it. The result is weakened, more brittle bones that can lead to fractures, rounded shoulders or shrinking height. It affects 25 million Americans, 80 percent of which are women. Those with arthritis are at greater risk for osteoporosis because of certain medications such as corticosteroids, which can reduce bone mass. Treatments include increasing calcium and vitamin D, medications, and weight-bearing exercise like walking.

Lupus: Lupus is a rheumatic disease – a disease involving the immune or musculoskeletal system – that affects skin, tissues and possibly organs. Women are eight to ten times more likely to get it than men are, and African Americans, Asians and Latinos more often than Caucasians. Symptoms can include a rash, sun sensitivity and inflammation of joints. It can be treated with medication for inflammation or to lower the immune system's activity; rest, exercise and diet.

Gout: Gout results from an excess of uric acid in the blood. The uric acid forms crystals that wind up in the joints (particularly in the big toe, ankles and knees), causing painful inflammation. Gout can be hereditary or result from excess consumption of alcohol or foods high in uric acid like liver, red meat, gravies, shellfish and some legumes. It can also be caused by obesity and some drugs used to treat high-blood pressure. It can be treated with medication and change in diet.

Back pain: Strain, injury or arthritis can trigger back pain that can range from mild to debilitating. Fifty to 80 percent of adults experience back pain at some point during their lives. Treatments include pain relievers, exercise, heat or cold packs, and learning self-protective habits.

Bursitis and tendinitis: Bursitis is inflammation of the bursa, a small sac filled with fluid that lies between the muscles and tendons or the muscles and bones. Tendinitis is inflammation of the tendon, the tissue that attaches muscles to bones. Although the cause is often hard to pinpoint, both conditions can be caused by overuse or injury, by poor posture or odd joint position, or as the result of other conditions – or even an infection. To treat the conditions, doctors recommend anti-inflammatories, heat or cold packs, and rest.

COMMON SYMPTOMS OF ARTHRITIS

Each condition has its own symptoms. But common to many forms of arthritis are inflamed and painful joints, stiffness, and even swelling. The symptoms can come and go, in many or single spots, and symptoms can appear whether you've been moving about or inactive. In some forms of arthritis, the skin over the painful spot may redden and feel warm. And some forms of arthritis are also associated with fatigue.

COMMON MEDICAL TREATMENTS FOR ARTHRITIS

Of course, many types of arthritis have resulted in many types of treatments. But below are some common ones.

Analgesics: Doctors often prescribe over-the-counter analgesics, or pain relievers, like acetaminophen (*Tylenol)* to reduce arthritis pain.

NSAIDs: For pain and swelling, physicians may prescribe anti-inflammatories called NSAIDs, which can cause stomach pain. If they do, stop taking them and call your doctor.

Biologic agents: Prescription drugs may also include biologic agents – drugs that target specific parts of the immune system to lower pain and inflammation.

Corticosteroids: Drugs called corticosteroids (sometimes called glucocorticoids), such as prednisone, may be given in pill form or as injections to reduce pain and inflammation. These can cause serious side effects such as suppressing the immune system or shifting fluids in the body. Anyone taking them needs close medical supervision.

Disease-modifiying antirheumatic drugs (DMARDs): DMARDs such as sulfasalazine and methotrexate slow down the progress of rheumatoid arthritis and some other types of inflammatory arthritis by suppressing the immune system. The prescription drugs can take weeks or months to work, and increase the risk of infections.

Sleep medications: Seventy-five percent of those with arthritis suffer from sleep difficulty, according to the National Sleep Foundation. Sleep medications like zolpidem (*Ambien*) or zaleplon (*Sonata*) can deepen sleep and help relax muscles. Doctors also sometimes prescribe a low-dose antidepressant, which can improve sleep, pain and depression.

Surgery: Surgery for arthritis is becoming more common, particularly arthroplasty or total joint replacement. Damaged joints are replaced by artificial components that can provide improved mobility and reduced pain. In some cases, operations such as synovectomies, osteotomies and arthrodeses are also performed to remove damaged portions of the joint or to reshape bone for pain relief and improved mobility.

The A-Z Guide

How to Use this Book

FOR PEOPLE WITH ARTHRITIS AND CAREGIVERS

The pages after this one list a range of alternative treatments in alphabetical order. Each entry will contain:

- The official name of the treatment
- Its common uses
- Scientific evidence
- Side effects and interactions
- Safety concerns
- Dosage, or ways to find a practitioner (whichever is applicable)

Under "scientific evidence," we list the names of the scientific or medical journal where the studies appeared. In some cases, the evidence suggests that a therapy is not safe. Those therapies will be marked by an icon warning 🔯. But whether a treatment is marked with a warning or not, it's important to talk with your doctor about any treatment you plan to try beforehand. He can recommend the appropriate dosage and talk to you about any side effects you might experience, about possible interactions with drugs you are already taking, and about any risks of the treatment. He can also help you assess when to stop a treatment that doesn't appear to be working. Your pharmacist can also be helpful in answering your questions and suggesting brands.

The information contained in this book is not intended to replace the advice of your medical doctor. As many of these treatments have not been approved by the U.S. Food and Drug Administration as arthritis therapies, we strongly urge you to consult your physician for guidance before trying any alternative or complementary treatment.

Ultimately, the decision to try an alternative treatment is up to you – as is the research and decision about where the treatment fits with your current treatment plan and budget. We hope you find this book a helpful guide in that process.

FOR MEDICAL PROFESSIONALS:

As you know, alternative medicine is immensely popular. In 1997 (the last national survey that included spending statistics), Americans spent $36-$47 billion on complementary therapies. Research funding is on the rise as well. NCCAM alone funded research to the tune of $117.7 million in 2004, more than double the funding five years ago. Top medical schools like those at Harvard University and the University of North Carolina, Chapel Hill, are incorporating integrative medical programs as well.

Patients in chronic pain – like those with arthritis – are flocking to these treatments out of frustration and hope. Many, however, are afraid to mention this to you, for fear you'll disapprove. We urge you to use this book as a starting point for a conversation about therapies your patients may want to try.

The book lists alternative treatments alphabetically according to the most common name of the therapy, from A to Z. In their descriptions, we draw on the most up to date scientific studies and evidence we can find, and cite those for our readers. We warn them away from treatments that researchers have found dangerous, and where there is little evidence for efficacy, we say so. The book has been edited and reviewed by physicians. (The experts' names and affiliations are listed in the acknowledgements page at the front of the book.) And throughout, we urge patients first to check with you, their physician.

Symbol Key

Because alternative treatments encompass a wide range – from supplements and herbs to massage and acupuncture, below is a symbol key to help you distinguish one type from the other. There are also treatments best avoided, and we've created a symbol to help easily recognize those treatments we consider potentially dangerous.

 These treatments are herbs or supplements in natural, pill, capsule, tincture, cream or liquid form.

 These treatments involve manipulation of tissues or joints, movement therapy or mind-body healing.

 WARNING! These treatments may be dangerous, and you should avoid them.

A-c

5-HTP (5-Hydroxytryptophan)

Common uses:
For the treatment of depression, anxiety, fibromyalgia; also for weight management

Our bodies produce their own 5-HTP from the amino acid tryptophan found in poultry, fish, beef and dairy product. The precursor to the neurotransmitter serotonin, 5-HTP is thought to be a mood-enhancer that increases pain tolerance, aids sleep and reduces hunger. The supplement is made from seeds of an African plant named Griffonia simplicifolia. By boosting serotonin levels, the supplement has been used to treat depression and fibromyalgia, and other conditions linked to low serotonin levels.

5-HTP is not without controversy, however. In 1989, the FDA banned tryptophan due to several deaths related to the blood disorder EMS. The tryptophan had been contaminated during manufacture. In 1998, the FDA confirmed that some 5-HTP products also had impurities.

5-HTP may also interact with some drugs and supplements so it's important to check with your doctor before using.

Scientific Evidence

Since the 1970s a number of small studies have shown that 5-HTP is effective in treating depression. However, reviews of the studies have been cautious, suggesting that

5-HTP may have had some effect but not enough to match that of traditional antidepressants. Others felt the studies were too small or lacking in controls to be definitive. In fact, a 2002 review of 108 studies concluded they were not sufficient to prove that 5-HTP was an effective treatment for depression.[Aust. NZ J Psychiatry. 2002 Aug; 36 (4): 499-91.]

Several recent studies, however, have shown 5-HTP to help relieve symptoms of panic, particularly in women. [J Psychopharmacol. 2004 Jun; 18 (2): 194-9.] [Psychiatry Res. 2002 Dec 30; 113 (3): 237-43.]

Several studies have also indicated that 5-HTP may be helpful in treating fibromyalgia. In one placebo-controlled study, for example, 50 patients were given 100 mg of 5-HTP three times a day for 90 days. Fifty percent of the patients showed significant improvement throughout the study. [J Int Med Res. 1992 Apri; 20(2): 182-9.]

A group of small Italian studies in the late '80s and '90s also suggest that 5-HTP is an effective weight-loss tool, suppressing carbohydrate cravings. Twenty-five obese patients with diabetes received 750 mg of 5-HTP or a placebo for two weeks. Those taking the 5-HTP cut back on carbohydrates and fat in particular and lost a significant amount of weight. [Int J Obes Relat Metab Disorder. 1998 Jul; 22 (7): 648-54.]

A few studies have also suggested that 5-HTP can improve sleep and migraines but more research is needed.

SIDE EFFECTS AND INTERACTIONS

- May include nausea, constipation, gas, drowsiness, or reduced sex drive.

- Combining 5-HTP with antidepressants; other psychiatric medications; over-the-counter cold medications (or any containing ephedrine or pseudophedrine); or medications for Parkinson's disease may cause anxiety, confusion and other serious side effects.

- Taken with antihistamines, muscle relaxants or narcotic pain relievers may increase drowsiness.

SAFETY CONCERNS

- In 1998, peak X, one of the impurities associated with the tryptophan deaths in 1989, was also founds in some 5-HTP products. The FDA believes that peak X may lead to the blood disorder EMS.

- Manufacturers remain responsible for screening for peak X and any other contaminants. But the FDA has not issued any more warnings about 5-HTP.

- If you do take 5-HTP, do so only under doctor supervision. Ask him to check your blood for elevated eosinophil levels (white blood cells whose rise could signal EMS).

DOSAGE

Start with 50 mg three times a day at mealtime to minimize side effects. If you have not experienced side effects after one week, raise the amount to 100 mg at each meal.

Acupressure

Common uses:
To relieve pain and stress, and improve well-being.

A form of bodywork that involves using the fingers, knuckles and palms to apply pressure along the body, acupressure has been practiced in China for 5,000 years. According to Chinese medicine, qi (pronounced chee), the body's energy, runs along fourteen pathways in the body called meridians. If one of the pathways or channels is blocked the result is pain or illness. Acupressure is thought to restore the flow of energy along the meridians. Some studies suggest that acupressure also releases endorphins, the body's natural painkillers.

SCIENTIFIC EVIDENCE

Although studies have been small, most suggest that acupressure can relieve nausea and pain. A 2002 Swedish study of 410 women undergoing gynecological surgery found that postoperative nausea was significantly reduced in the acupressure groups compared to the control group. [Can J Anaesth. 2002 Dec; 49 (10): 1034-9.] A 2004 Taiwanese study of 146 people treated for chronic low back pain found acupressure more effective than physical therapy. [Prev Med. 2004 Jul; 39 (1): 168-76.] And in a clinical trial, those treated with acupressure over eight weeks (preceded by acupoint stimulation) had 39 percent less lower back pain than the control group at the end of the treatments. [Complement Ther Med. 2004 Mar;12(1):28-37.]

SAFETY CONCERNS

- Acupressure is considered safe – although acupressurists are not required to be licensed. Some are certified through the National Certification Commission for Acupuncture and Oriental Medicine (NCCAOM). Once you do find a practitioner, ask if he has a certificate from an acupressure school.

- A practitioner should never press an open wound, swollen or inflamed skin, bruises, surgical scars, varicose veins, broken bones, lymph nodes or tumors.

- You should not have acupressure if you have a contagious condition, or a heart, kidney or lung disorder.

- Tell your practitioner if you are pregnant so that she can avoid certain acupressure points.

FINDING AN ACUPRESSURIST

Ask your doctor for a referral. The following organization also offers a referral list.

- American Organization for Bodywork Therapies of Asia
  (856) 782 1616
  www.aobta.org

Acupuncture

Common uses:

To treat low back and myofascial pain; pain from headaches, migraines, menstrual cramps, fibromyalgia, osteoarthritis or dental work; nausea caused by pregnancy, anesthesia or chemotherapy; asthma, infertility, carpal tunnel syndrome and addiction.

Acupuncture has been practiced throughout Asia for thousands of years. Like acupressure, it's based on the theory that qi – considered in Oriental medicinal philosophy to be the body's life energy – flows through the body along lines called meridians. Illness like arthritis can cause an imbalance in qi, and out-of-balance qi can cause illness or pain. Very fine needles inserted into the skin along the meridians can correct the flow of qi, restoring balance and blocking pain. Although Western scientists aren't sure why acupuncture works, they believe that it may stimulate the central nervous system, which in turn releases endorphins or other chemicals in the brain that block pain.

SCIENTIFIC EVIDENCE

In 1997, after evaluating hundreds of acupuncture studies, the National Institutes of Health determined that acupuncture is effective for postoperative pain after dental surgery, and to treat nausea from chemotherapy, pregnancy and anesthesia. It also found acupuncture a helpful treatment for a number of conditions including fibromyalgia, headaches and carpal tunnel syndrome. A 2004 review of clinical trials drew similar conclusions. [J Altern Complement. Med. 2004 June; 10 (3): 468-80.] A 2002 Brazilian study showed that the treatment of fibromyalgia with acupuncture reduced pain and depression. [Rheumawire 11/22/02]. Several 2004 studies point specifically to acupuncture's efficacy in treating osteoarthritis. In a three-year Spanish study of 563 patients with osteoarthritis of the knee, for example, 75 percent had a 45 percent reduction in pain with weekly treatments. [Acupunct Med. 2004; 22 (1):23-8.]

SAFETY CONCERNS

- Acupuncture is considered safe if it is done by a licensed practitioner with sterilized, disposable needles.

- The practitioner should use needles from a sealed package and should swab the puncture site with alcohol first. Otherwise, you could be at risk for infection.

- Consult your physician before deciding on acupuncture.

- Your acupuncturist should take a medical history before treatment. Be sure to tell him about any medications or supplements you take. Also tell him if you have a pacemaker, breast implants or are pregnant.

FINDING AN ACUPUNCTURIST

Ask your doctor for a referral. You can also check with the following organizations:

- The American Academy of Medical Acupuncture Offers a list of medical doctors who practice acupuncture.
  (323) 937-5514
  www.medicalacupuncture.org

- Acupuncture and Oriental Medicine Alliance (AOM Alliance) Refers visitors to state-licensed or national board certified acupuncturists
  (253) 851-6896
  www.aomalliance.org

- National Certification Commission for Acupuncture and Oriental Medicine (NCCAOM) Offers list of certified practitioners.
  (703) 548-9004
  www.nccaom.org

- American Association of Oriental Medicine lists practitioners by location.
  (916) 451-6950
  www.aaom.org

Alexander Technique

Common uses:

Corrects poor posture, which in turn reduces muscle tension and increases ease of movement.

The movement technique, founded in 1896 by Frederick Matthias Alexander, an Australian actor, addresses poor posture in order to increase ease of movement and diminish muscle tension. The idea behind the method is that proper alignment of the head, neck and spine improves health. AT is taught one on one or in a group sessions that last about 45 minutes. The instructor observes how you walk, stand, sit, bend and lie down, and then corrects your posture through instruction and touch.

SCIENTIFIC EVIDENCE

Scientific studies on the technique are scant. A 1999 study showed that AT improved balance in healthy older women. [J Gerontol A Biol Sci Med Sci. 1999 Jan; 54 (1): M8-11.] A 2003 review of controlled clinical trials found only two that were sound in method and that had clinically relevant results, indicating that the techniques reduced disability in those with Parkinson's disease and with back pain. [Forsch Komplementarmed Klass Naturheilkd. 2003 Dec; 10 (6): 325-9.] A 2002 British study of 93 people with Parkinson's disease showed that AT improved movement ease and lifted depression significantly more than in the massage group or control group. [Clinical Rehabilitation 2002; 16: 705-718] Another study found that in conjunction with other therapies, AT could reduce back pain. [Clin Exp Reheumatol 1996 May-Jun; 14 (3): 281]

SAFETY CONCERNS

- AT is safe even for pregnant women provided it is taught by a qualified instructor.
- If a position causes pain, stop.

FINDING AN AT INSTRUCTOR

Check with your physician or local practitioners. You can also check with the following organizations.

- American Society for the Alexander Technique offers a three-year certification course and referral service
  (800) 473-0620 or (413) 584-2359
  www.alexandertech.org

- The American Center for the Alexander Technique, Inc. also offers a three-year certification program and teacher referral service.
  (212) 633-2229
  www.acatnyc.org

Aloe Vera

Common uses:
Applied topically, aloe vera reduces inflammation and aids healing of burns and scrapes. Taken internally, it's used to treat rheumatoid arthritis and as a laxative.

Aloe vera belongs to the lily family and grows wild in Madagascar and Africa. It's also grown commercially in the United States, Japan, the Caribbean and Mediterranean. It's best known for the healing clear gel inside its leaves used to treat burns, scrapes, shingles and psoriasis. Aloe vera juice may relieve heartburn and ulcers. Another part, aloe vera latex from the leaf skin, is dried into a powder and used as a laxative.

SCIENTIFIC EVIDENCE

A number of studies show that aloe vera lessens inflammation. For instance, in a 1989 study, mice that received aloe vera both in their drinking water and topically healed more quickly than the control group. [J Am Podiatr Med Assoc. 1989 Nov; 79 (11): 559-62.] Mice receiving 100 and 300 mg of aloe vera daily for four days blocked substances that interfere with wound healing. [J Am Podiatr Med Assoc. 1994 Dec; 84 (12): 614.21.] Rats whose burns were treated with aloe vera gel had less inflammation and more healing than control groups after both 7 and 14 days. [J Med Assoc Thai. 2000 Apr; 83 (4): 417-25.] A double-blind trial of a laxative containing aloe vera showed it was an effective laxative compared with the control group. [Digest 49:65-71,1991.]

SIDE EFFECTS AND INTERACTIONS

- Long-term use of laxatives, including aloe vera latex, can cause potassium loss, a mineral that helps maintain fluid balance and is essential for the transmission of nerve impulses. It's especially dangerous if you are already taking a diuretic, corticosteroids or a digitalis heart medication.

- Aloe vera may slow healing on deep wounds.

- Taken internally, aloe vera may increase the effects of several drugs, including corticosteroids.

- Topical use may sometimes cause a rash. If so, stop using.

- The juice can sometimes contain aloe latex, causing cramps, diarrhea or loose stools. If so, throw it away.

SAFETY CONCERNS

- Read the label on any product to make sure that aloe vera is one of the first ingredients listed. Otherwise, you may be getting a diluted product. Creams and gels should contain at least 20 percent aloe vera.

- Make certain that aloe juice is not derived from aloe latex and that it does not contain aloin or aloe-emoin compounds, substances in aloe latex.

- Drink aloe juice between meals. Otherwise it may interfere with the absorption of nutrients, and the food may decrease the absorption of the aloe vera.

- Make sure that aloe vera juice has an IASC-certified seal, which indicates that it has been processed according to the standards of the International Aloe Science Council.

- Do not inject aloe vera. In 1998 several cancer patients injected with aloe vera died.

- During pregnancy, aloe vera can cause uterine contractions and miscarriage.

- Do not use aloe latex laxative when pregnant, breast-feeding or menstruating. It can trigger uterine contractions.

- Aloe vera for internal use should be pasteurized and contain preservatives to prevent contamination.

- If the leaf products of aloe vera aren't separated properly, the gel can contain a purgative called anthraquinones, which, ingested, can cause intestinal pain and damage.

- Do not give children or elderly, or anyone with intestinal difficulty aloe vera latex.

DOSAGE

- For burns, sunburns and shingles, apply as needed.

- For cuts and scrapes, apply cream or gel two to three times a day.

- For heartburn, drink two ounces four times daily.

- For insect bites, apply gel four times a day.

- For ulcers, drink one half cup twice a day for one month.

Aromatherapy

Common uses:
To relieve stress and promote a feeling of well-being.

People have used essential oils from trees, plants and herbs to treat various conditions for centuries. But it was a French chemist, Rene-Maurice Gattefosse, who coined the term in 1928 after he noticed the effectiveness of essential oils when treating wounds in World War I. Today aromatherapists use about fifty oils to treat conditions from stress to muscle tightness. (Rosemary oil is thought to relieve pain and help relax muscles.) The oils can be mixed with a neutral vegetable oil for use in a massage; they can be inhaled; or they can be added to bathwater. It's easy to do aromatherapy at home or go to an aromatherapist who can mix several oils to address a specific condition.

SCIENTIFIC EVIDENCE

Research indicates that the oils activate the olfactory nerve cells in the nasal cavity, which then send messages to the limbic system of the brain associated with emotions and memory. They may also help relieve certain conditions by stimulating the immune, circulatory or nervous systems. In a British study of 122 patients in an intensive care unit, those receiving aromatherapy reported better moods and less anxiety than those receiving massage or bed rest. [Journal of Advanced Nursing (England) Jan 1995, 21 (1) p. 34-40] A 2004 study of 90 college women given lavender, neroli (oil from a bitter orange tree) or a placebo found that the relaxing odor of lavender led to lowered heart rate and skin moisture, and that the stimulating odor of neroli accomplished the reverse. [Psychol Rep. 2004 Jun; 94 (3 Pt 2): 1127-36.] A small study of 26 men and women found that their pain diminished after treatment with lavender. [Psychosom Med. 2004 Jul-Aug; 66 95): 599-606.]

SIDE EFFECTS AND INTERACTIONS

- Some oil can cause allergic skin rashes. If that happens, try a different oil.

- Don't mix soap and oil in a bath. The soap may interfere with the absorption of the oil.

SAFETY CONCERNS

- Essential oils are for external use only.

- Certain oils can trigger bronchial spasms. If you have asthma, speak to your doctor before using any oil.

- Avoid during pregnancy. Some oils can harm the fetus if taken internally or even if applied externally.

- Aromatherapy is not a substitute for traditional medical care.

FINDING AN AROMATHERAPIST

Aromatherapists are not licensed in the United States. The best way to find one is to ask your doctor or another licensed practitioner for a referral. Or find a licensed practitioner of another therapy like massage who also does aromatherapy. You can also contact The National Association for Holistic Aromatherapy (NAHA), (206) 547-2164, www.naha.org.

Avocado/Soybean Oil (ASU)

Common uses:

To help relieve pain of osteoarthritis.

Theoretically, the mixture of one third avocado oil and two thirds soybean oil helps relieve the pain of osteoarthritis by inhibiting cartilage destruction and by stimulating its repair. ASU has been used in France as a prescription treatment for osteoarthritis for more than 15 years as Piascledine 300. That brand is not available in the United States but ASU is sold here as a supplement.

SCIENTIFIC EVIDENCE

In a 1998 French double-blind, placebo-controlled study of 164 people with severe osteoarthritis of the knee or hip, half received 300 mg of ASU for six months. Both groups improved but the group taking the oil had significantly less pain and disability than the placebo group. [Arthritis & Rheum 1998;41:81-91.] In a similar three-month double-blind study, ASU reduced the need for treatment with NSAID, or anti-inflammatories, in 164 patients with knee or hip osteoarthritis. [Curr Rheumatol Rep 2000;2:472-7] Two combined studies showed that ASU lessened disability, pain and dependence on NSAIDs in those with osteoarthritis. [Cochrane Database Syst Rev 2001; http://www.update-software.com/abstracts/ab002947.htm3; accessed November 10, 2003.]

SIDE EFFECTS AND INTERACTIONS

• Some people may have mild gastrointestinal discomfort.

SAFETY CONCERNS

• Do not buy products that say "Avocado and/or Soy Oil." That is not the same thing as ASU.

DOSAGE

300 mg capsule once a day.

Ayurveda

Common uses:

To address energy imbalances in the body, mind and spirit, particularly stress-related conditions such as chronic fatigue syndrome, fibromyalgia, irritable bowel syndrome.

Ayurveda is a complete medical system practiced in India for more than 5,000 years. The name means science of life, and its approach is largely preventive. The practice is based on the belief that every individual contains life energy called prana, and the five elements: earth, air, fire, water and space. The elements combine into three types of energy, or doshas: vata, pitta and kapha. Illness is caused by imbalance in one or more of the doshas. By applying ayurvedic practices involving vegetarian diet, exercise, meditation, herbal treatments, breathing and purification techniques, a person's doshas can be rebalanced.

In the West, Ayurveda practices are often used to address conditions that may be affected by stress such as chronic fatigue syndrome, fibromyalgia and irritable bowel syndrome.

SCIENTIFIC EVIDENCE

Although many individual aspects of Ayurveda have been studied, its practice has a whole has not been carefully evaluated, at least not by standards acceptable to Western scientists. Meditation, yoga and breathing exercises, however, are widely accepted as healthy practices as is the emphasis on exercise and a diet full of fresh fruits and vegetables. Researchers are currently investigating the effect of Ayurvedic medicine on cancer, asthma, peri-menopausal symptoms, premenstrual syndrome, painful menstruation (dysmenorrhea), the immune system, cholesterol, hypertension, herpes, depression and diabetes.

SIDE EFFECTS AND INTERACTIONS

- Following an Ayurvedic diet may interfere with diets recommended for heart disease and diabetes.

- Some herbal preparations can interact with other medications. Check with your doctor.

SAFETY CONCERNS

- Those with serious chronic illness like heart disease or diabetes should not rely on Ayurvedic medicine alone.

- Cleansing with laxatives or enemas – both Ayurvedic practices – can cause chemical imbalances. Check with your doctor first. Make sure that any equipment used in such cleansings is sterile.

- If you are on a special diet because of heart disease or diabetes, consult your doctor before starting Ayurvedic diet practices.

- Consult your doctor before taking any herbal preparations. And tell your Ayurvedic practitioner what medications you are taking.

FINDING AN AYURVEDIC PRACTITIONER

The United States does not offer licensing for Ayurvedic practitioners although U.S. Ayurvedic centers do offer one-year training programs (the programs in India are five and a half years or longer).

Ideally, opt for a practitioner who has a degree in Ayurvedic medicine from a qualified Ayurvedic university in India. The following organizations offer information and referrals.

- The National Institute of Ayurvedic Medicine
  (845) 278-8700
  www.niam.com.

- The Maharishi College of Vedic Medicine
  (505) 830-0415 or (800) 811-0550
  www.mcvmnm.org

Balneotherapy

Balneotherapy is the use of warm water and minerals (or mineral-rich mud) to reduce stiffness and pain. See hydrotherapy on p. 138.

Bee Venom Therapy

Common uses:

Used as an anti-inflammatory for conditions such as tendinitis, bursitis, rheumatoid arthritis and osteoarthritis.

The use of bee venom therapy can be traced to ancient times, when even Hippocrates, the Greek physician, used bee venom to treat arthritis and other joint problems. A Vermont beekeeper popularized the therapy in the United States sixty years ago. The practice involves administering bee venom by injection or via a bee sting. The venom contains anti-inflammatories called adolapin and melittin, which stimulate the production of cortisol, a natural steroid.

SCIENTIFIC EVIDENCE

A 2004 study of mice with induced arthritis showed that after eight weeks of bee venom injections the incidence of arthritis was significantly lower than in the control group. [Am J Chin Med. 2004; 32 (3): 361-7.] In a 2002 study of rats with induced arthritis, bee venom injections suppressed the inflammation caused by arthritis. [Am J Chin Med. 2002; 30 (1): 73-80.] In a very small study of five multiple sclerosis patients treated bee venom at Georgetown University Medical Center, three felt increased strength or decreased pain.

SIDE EFFECTS AND INTERACTIONS

- Bee stings can be painful and may not work. If you see no improvement after eight sessions and a total of 20-70 stings or injections, it's probably not going to work for you.

SAFETY CONCERNS

- Do not use if you are allergic to bee venom. Keep a bee-venom allergy kit (with syringe and epinephrine) handy in case you turn out to be allergic.

- Do not use bee venom if you have heart disease, hypertension, tuberculosis or diabetes.

DOSAGE

Some people find relief after several sessions; others go back every several months for additional shots.

FINDING A PRACTITIONER

Bee venom injections are only FDA approved for desensitizing those with bee allergies. If you do find a physician who will administer venom, he probably won't charge you for the venom. The best way to find a physician who uses bee venom is word-of-mouth or through a pain clinic. To find a beekeeper who applies bee stings, contact the American Apitherapy Society, (914) 725-7944; www.apitherapy.org. Do not try the procedure on your own.

Biofeedback

Common uses:

Biofeedback is used to control chronic pain, stress, anxiety, muscle tension and gastrointestinal disorders.

Biofeedback combines electronic technology and mind-body techniques to teach people to regulate autonomic body functions such as blood pressure, pulse and muscle tension. A physician places sensors on the part of the body he will monitor and attaches those to electronic equipment that displays the body responses such as skin temperature, heart rates, and brain waves. The patient then learns mind-body techniques such as visualization or relaxation to influence those responses, lowering heart rate or relaxing muscles for example. The goal is to teach the patient to be able to monitor and make those changes on his own. The number of sessions needed varies from several to 20, depending on how long it takes to learn to effect and control responses.

SCIENTIFIC EVIDENCE

A number of small studies suggest that biofeedback can be effective in reducing arthritic and other kinds of pain. For example, in a 1997 German study, 18 patients with fibromyalgia received nine biofeedback treatments over four weeks. The result was a significant reduction in pain intensity and increased muscular sensitivity. [Percept Mot Skills. 1997 Jun; 84 (3 PT l): 1043-50.] In a 1992 study of 8 children with rheumatoid arthritis, 50 to 62 percent had less pain immediately following a six-session treatment that involved relaxation training, electromyograms (measurement of muscle electrical activity) and biofeedback. Sixty-two to 88 percent had a 25 percent reduction in pain after six months. [Arthritis Care Research 1992 June; 5 (2): 101-10.] There are also studies suggesting improvement in a number of conditions such as Raynaud's phenomenon, scleroderma, lupus and stress.

Side Effects and Interactions

None

Safety Concerns

- If you wear a pacemaker or have a serious heart disorder, consult your doctor before using biofeedback.

- If you are diabetic and using biofeedback to control your circulation, monitor your blood sugar for possible changes.

- Ask your doctor to recommend what brand of biofeedback equipment to purchase for home use.

Finding a Practitioner

It's best to get a referral from your doctor to a certified professional. Regulations and certification requirements vary by state. Many practitioners are certified by the Biofeedback Certification Institute of America, which also provides referrals: (303) 420-2902 or www.bcia.org.

Bitter Melon/Bitterin Oil

Common uses:

The melon is used to lower blood sugar and cholesterol, and to treat cancer, viral infections, and immune disorders. The oil is used topically to relieve inflammation and to treat wounds.

Bitter melon is grown in tropical parts of Asia, East Africa, and South America. Practitioners of Chinese medicine have used it to treat diabetes for hundreds of years. Some believe it also lowers cholesterol. The oil is used to treat wounds and as an anti-inflammatory.

SCIENTIFIC EVIDENCE

The bulk of evidence surrounds the use of bitter melon for diabetes. A 2003 review of studies to date by Harvard Medical School concluded the results regarding bitter melon (and a number of other herbs and dietary supplements viewed separately) and diabetes were positive but preliminary. [Diabetes Care. 2003 Apr;26(4):1277-94.] Another Indian review noted that over 100 studies have authenticated its use for diabetes and its complications, and as an antibacterial and antiviral treatment as well. The studies have also shown its effectiveness against some cancers. [J Ethnopharmacol. 2004 Jul;93(1):123-32.] A 1986 study of 18 adult diabetics showed a 20 to 30 percent reduction in blood sugar after taking bitter melon. [Ethnopharmacol 1986; 17: 227-82] In vitro and animal studies show some antiviral activity against HIV, herpes, and some protective effects against leukemia and breast cancer.

SIDE EFFECTS AND INTERACTIONS

- Excessive dosages may cause abdominal pain, diarrhea, headache or fever. It should not be used with insulin or hypoglycemic drugs.

Safety Concerns

- Consult your doctor before using it if you are diabetic, hyperglycemic, pregnant or nursing.

Dosage

Puree the fruit (found in Asian groceries) with an equal amount of water. Drink ¼ to ½ cup a day. If you buy bitter melon juice, take ¼ to ½ cup of that. And if you take an extract, take ¼ to ½ teaspoon per day.

Boron

Common uses:

To treat osteoarthritis and osteoporosis; improve memory, regulate hormones, and help the body metabolize magnesium.

Boron is a trace mineral that helps the body use calcium and magnesium. It may also help prevent bone loss and improve bone and joint health. Boron is found in fruits like apples, pears, and grapes; vegetables, nuts and dried beans.

Scientific Evidence

Studies of large populations indicate that in areas of the world where the intake of boron is one mg a day or less, the range of arthritis is 20 to 70 percent. In populations which get 3 to 10 mg of boron a day, the incidence is far less, about zero to 10 percent. [Environ Health Perspect. 1994 Nov;102 Suppl 7:83-5.] In a 1996 British study, researchers found that bone close to arthritic joints had significantly lower concentrations of boron than normal joints. [Bone. 1996 Feb; 18 (2): 151-7.] A small British study showed that boron aids those with osteoarthritis. [Journal of Nutritional Medicine. Vol.1.Abingdon, Oxfordshire. U.K.: Carfax, 1990: 127-32.]

SIDE EFFECTS AND INTERACTIONS

- May cause diarrhea and upset stomach.

- May irritate skin, mouth, eyes and throat.

- May increase levels of calcium in the blood, especially if you are already taking supplements containing calcium.

SAFETY CONCERNS

- Excessive doses can be poisonous.

- Boron may increase estrogen levels, which could up the risk of cancer in some women. It should not be taken with birth control pills, hormonal replacement therapy or any drugs containing estrogen.

- Those with an allergy to boric acid, borax, citrate, aspartate or glycinate should not take boron.

- Pregnant and nursing women should avoid boron.

DOSAGE

Doses of 3 to 6 mg a day have been used in studies. You may already get 3 mg of boron from your diet and/or from a multivitamin, so you should not take more than three additional mg a day. Calcium supplements often contain boron so be sure to read the label.

Boswellia

Common uses:
Boswellia is used to treat osteoarthritis, rheumatoid arthritis, asthma, bladder inflammation and inflammatory bowel diseases like Crohn's disease and ulcerative colitis.

Boswellia comes from the Boswellia serrata tree in India. Its resin, oil and gum have been used for centuries by Ayurvedic practitioners to treat inflammation. Today it's available in pill, cream or extract form to reduce inflammation of osteoarthritis and rheumatoid arthritis. It's also used to treat menstrual pain and to soothe bruises and sores.

SCIENTIFIC EVIDENCE

Research suggests that the acids in boswellia keep inflammatory white cells form entering damaged tissue and improve blood flow to the joints. The acids also inhibit something called leukotriene synthesis, a contributor to inflammation. In a small 1998, double-blind German study, 70 percent of patients with asthma given 300 mgs of boswellia three times daily for six weeks improved dramatically. [Eur J Med Res. 1998 Nov 17; 3 (11): 511-4.] In a 2003 double-blind Indian study of 30 patients with osteoarthritis of the knee, those receiving boswellia extract for eight weeks reported decreased knee pain and increased function. [Phytomedicine. 003 Jan; 10 (1): 3-7]. However, in a 1998 double-blind German study, boswellia had no measurable effect on patients with rheumatoid arthritis. [Z Rheumatol. 1998 Feb; 57 (1): 11-6.]

SIDE EFFECTS AND INTERACTIONS

- May cause nausea, acid reflux, diarrhea, and skin rash

- It may increase the effects of cholesterol-lowering and anti-cancer drugs, and of supplements like glucosamine and chondroitin used to treat joint disease.

- It may lessen the effect of anti-inflammatories like ibuprofen (*Advil*, *Motrin*, *Nuprin*), aspirin and naproxen sodium (*Aleve*).

SAFETY CONCERNS

- May cause spontaneous abortion in pregnant women. Lactating women should not use it either.

- Boswellia in children may mask asthma symptoms.

- Don't take boswellia for more than 12 weeks and don't exceed the recommended dosage.

DOSAGE

150 mg three times a day.

Bromelain

Common uses:

Used for muscle aches, arthritis, heartburn and aiding digestion.

Bromelain is an enzyme found in pineapple that works as an anti-inflammatory and blood thinner by breaking down fibrin, a blood-clotting protein that can interfere with circulation and keep tissues from draining properly. Bromelain also blocks the production of compounds that can cause swelling and pain.

SCIENTIFIC EVIDENCE

A number of studies highlight bromelain's anti-inflammatory effect. A 1995 German open study of people with strains and torn ligaments showed they had significantly less pain and swelling after taking bromelain than those taking NSAIDs. [Fortsch Med 1995 Jul 10; 113 (19): 303]. In a 2002 open British study of 77 subjects with knee pain given either 200 or 400 mg doses of bromelain, all the symptoms were significantly reduced, more so in the group on a higher dose. [Phytomedicine. 2002 Dec; 9 (8): 681-6.] However in a 2002 double-blind study at Indiana State University, subjects taking bromelain or ibuprofen for muscle soreness showed no difference in relief than those taking a placebo or nothing. [Clin J Sport Med 2002 Nov; 12 (6): 373-8.] A review of studies also concluded that bromelain is effective at fighting tumor cells. [Cell Mol Life Sci.2001 Aug; 58 (9): 1234-45.]

SIDE EFFECTS AND INTERACTIONS

- Large doses can cause upset stomach, diarrhea, excess menstrual bleeding or skin rash. People with ulcers should not take bromelain.

- Do not take if you are allergic to pineapple.

- Bromelain may increase the risk of bleeding when used with anticoagulants such as heparin or warfarin (*Coumadin*), aspirin and other NSAIDs. That's also true if used with supplements that increase the risk of bleeding such as gingko biloba or garlic.
- It may increase the effect of tetracycline, an antibiotic.

SAFETY CONCERNS

None

DOSAGE

Enzymes are measured in GDUs (gelatin digesting units) or MCUs (milk clotting units). The amount of those in a milligram dose may vary. And one GDU equals 1.5 MCU. Dose suggestions range from 4,000 GDU (6,000 MCU) to 6,000 GDU (9,000 MCU). Take it on an empty stomach if you are using it as an anti-inflammatory. Take just before eating if you are using it for indigestion or heartburn.

Burdock Root

Common uses:

To soothe chronic skin ailments, rheumatoid arthritis symptoms; to prevent cancer; also used as a diuretic, mild laxative, digestive aid, and a way to lower blood sugar.

Burdock is a carrot-like root vegetable popular in Japan. It's found in Asian grocery stores and some health-food stores. Brown-skinned with white flesh, it tastes similar to celery and artichokes when cooked and bitter when raw. Fifty percent of the vegetable is a carbohydrate called inulin. Inulin may be behind the vegetable's ability to lower blood sugar. It may also act as an anti-inflammatory and stimulate immune cells that help skin conditions such as eczema. It also may promote the growth of friendly bacteria in the intestines.

SCIENTIFIC EVIDENCE

There is little clinical evidence backing its uses. Studies in Germany (1967) and Japan (1986) suggest antibiotic effects. Several Korean studies suggest antioxidant effects. [Am J Chin Med. 1996; 24 (2): 127-37. [Am J Chin Med. 2000; 28 (2): 163-73.]

SIDE EFFECTS AND INTERACTIONS

- Compounds called glyosides stimulate the bowels and probably the uterus.

- May cause skin rash.

- Diabetics should consult with their doctors before using burdock.

SAFETY CONCERNS

- Animal studies suggest that burdock stimulates the uterus. Pregnant and nursing women should not eat burdock.

DOSAGE

Two to six grams of dried root daily, or three cups of dried burdock tea daily (one teaspoon dried root boiled in three cups of water for 30 minutes). Or 425-475 mg capsules 3 times per day.

Cat's Claw

Common uses:
Reduces inflammation and pain, and boosts the immune system.

Cat's claw comes from the inner bark of a vine that grows in Peru and Bolivia. The name comes from the cat-claw look of two thorns at the leaves' base. Amazonians have used cat's claw to treat any number of ailments from cancer to arthritis to skin conditions – and even contraception. But scientists are most interested in its anti-inflammatory and immune-boosting properties.

SCIENTIFIC EVIDENCE

In a study of 45 patients with osteoarthritis, those treated with cat's claw for four weeks had significantly reduced pain compared to those treated with placebo. [Inflamm Res. 2001; 50 (9): 442-8.] In a double blind trial, patients with rheumatoid arthritis given cat's claw for 52 weeks had a significant reduction in pain and swollen joints. [J Rheumatol. 2002 Apr.; 29 (4): 678-81.] Several in vitro studies have also shown cat's claw to be effective in reducing cancer cells.

SIDE EFFECTS AND INTERACTIONS

- May cause stomach upset, nausea, headache and dizziness.

- May increase the risk of bleeding when taken with anticoagulants such as heparin or warfarin (*Coumadin*), aspirin, NSAIDs, or supplements such as ginkgo, biloba, garlic or chamomile.

- May interfere with the way the liver breaks down some drugs and supplements. Consult your doctor before using.

- May slow heartbeats or lower blood pressure. Do no use if you are taking anti-hypertensive medication or drugs for irregular heart rhythms.

SAFETY CONCERNS

- Taken in high doses, it may cause diarrhea, bleeding gums, bruising and lowered blood pressure.

- A member of the acacia species grown in the Southwest is also called cat's claw and is poisonous. The two species used for treatments are Uncaria guianensis and Uncaria tomentosa.

- Women who are pregnant, breastfeeding or who wish to become pregnant should not use cat's claw.

- People with auto-immune disorders such as rheumatoid arthritis, lupus, multiple sclerosis, or HIV should consult their doctor before using cat's claw. It may overstimulate the immune system, worsening symptoms.

- Do not use if you have had or plan to have an organ or tissue transplant.

DOSAGE

In pill form, take 250 mg between meals twice a day.

As a tea, 1 to two teaspoons of the dried herb per cup, up to three times a day.

Cayenne or Red Pepper

Common uses:

Pain reliever, digestive aid

Cayenne is packed with capsaicin, a phytochemical that gives chilies their heat. Capsaicin is used as a painkiller in commercial creams to ease the pain of arthritis and shingles. It may work by interfering with substance P, a chemical that transmits pain signals. It also releases endorphins, the body's natural pain relievers. The capsaicin in chili peppers also increases the secretions of mucous, temporarily clearing congestion. And it's thought to aid digestion by increasing blood flow to the stomach and intestines, by stimulating digestive juices, and by inhibiting bacteria that may cause ulcers.

SCIENTIFIC EVIDENCE

A number of studies have shown capsaicin to be an effective pain reliever. For instance, in a double-blind study of 70 patients with osteoarthritis and 31 with rheumatoid arthritis, 80 percent of those treated with capsaicin cream had a reduction in pain after two weeks of treatments. [Clin Ther. 1991 May-June; 13 (3): 383-95.] When 96 arthritic patients applied capsaicin cream to arthritic joints for twelve weeks in a double-blind study, 81 percent of the patients had significantly fewer arthritic symptoms, including less morning stiffness, compared to only 54 percent of those using plain cream. [Seminars in Arthritis and Rheumatism, June '94; 23: Suppl 3: 25-33.] A number of studies also suggest that capsaicin protects the mucous lining in the intestines and helps to heal ulcers.

SIDE EFFECTS AND INTERACTIONS

- Discontinue if capsaicin irritates your skin.
- If you get it in your eyes or inside your nose, it will burn intensely but does no damage.
- Too many chilies may cause diarrhea and stomach pain.
- Capsaicin causes no problems when taken with drugs or herbs.

SAFETY CONCERNS

- Don't use on broken or irritated skin.
- Keep cayenne away from children.
- Don't use capsaicin and a heating pad or hot towel simultaneously; you'll increase the risk of burns.

DOSAGE

Use a dime-sized amount of topical cream on painful area. Leave on for at least 30 minutes.

Chinese Herbs

Common uses:

Because Chinese herbs are an integral part of Chinese medicine, they are used for any number of maladies from sinus congestion to arthritis to menopausal symptoms.

All Chinese herbs aren't exactly herbs. Most come from plants and vegetables but others are from minerals or animal products. Chinese herbs are primarily used in combinations of anything from two herbs to dozens. American researchers know little about Chinese herbs although some are beginning to be studied in the U.S. with positive results.

SCIENTIFIC EVIDENCE

In an Australian double-blind study, subjects with irritable bowel syndrome taking individualized herbal formulas had significantly more symptom relief after 16 weeks than did those taking placebos. [JAMA 1998' 280 (18): 1585-1589.] When 54 patients with rheumatoid arthritis were given acupuncture plus a Chinese herb, all 54 felt some relief. [J Tradit Chin Med (China) Sep 1993, 12 (3) p 174-8.] And when mice in which arthritis was induced were given a mixture of 12 herbs known as PG201, the progression of the arthritis was significantly reduced. [Rheumatology (Oxford). 2003 May; 42 (5): 665-72.] Some well-designed studies are under way in the U.S. and in China to evaluate the effectiveness of some Chinese herbs.

SIDE EFFECTS AND INTERACTIONS

- For the most part, it's not known if Chinese herbs are safe to take with conventional medicines.

SAFETY CONCERNS

- Ask an experienced practitioner for herbs or for a reputable source. Some herbal preparations have been contaminated with pesticides, metals or even other drugs.

- Consult a medical doctor before taking Chinese herbs.

- Long-term use of some herbs can affect the liver. Again, consult with your doctor.

- Some Chinese herbs are dangerous during pregnancy.

- Chinese herbs are regulated as "dietary supplements." The FDA has not evaluated their effectiveness or safety. However, the Chinese government is taking some steps to ensure their safety.

- If you feel nausea, stomach distress or tenderness, or have coughs or fever, stop taking the herbs immediately and call your doctor.

DOSAGE

The first rule: don't exceed the recommended dosage. Dosages vary from preparation to preparation. Chinese herbs can come as pills, potions or liniments.

Chinese Medicine

Common uses:
Preventing and treating illness; pain relief

Traditional Chinese medicine has been practiced in Asia for thousands of years. Some examples have already been covered (or will be covered) in this book – acupuncture, acupressure and Chinese herbal remedies, for example. The medical system is based on a belief in the balance of energies call yin and yang. Yin and yang are also called feminine and masculine, and each person contains some combination of those energies. To be healthy, the energies need to be balanced. Another source of energy is called qi (pronounced chee). Qi flows along meridians throughout the body. When qi is blocked, illness follows.

If you visit a Chinese medicine practitioner, he will look at the pattern of your symptoms rather than for a specific illness. Like a Western doctor, he will perform a physical exam and then offer a diagnosis based on your qi deficiency and then make suggestions for reestablishing balance that may include herbs, acupuncture, massage, and changes in diet and exercise.

SCIENTIFIC EVIDENCE

Studies on different aspects of Chinese medicine such as massage, acupuncture, have suggested their effectiveness. Acupuncture for instance can be helpful in easing the pain of arthritis. (See p. 41) Certain forms of gentle exercise like tai chi and qi gong may also help improve balance and ease of movement. (See p. 226) And research on the effectiveness of Chinese herbs is increasing in the United States and in China. (See Chinese herbs above.)

SIDE EFFECTS AND INTERACTIONS

- Some herbs may interact with other drugs. Check with your doctor before using them.

SAFETY CONCERNS

- Talk to your doctor before seeing a Chinese medicine practitioner. And make certain that whatever practitioner you see is certified and experienced.

- If you have acupuncture, make sure the practitioner uses sterile, disposable needles.

FINDING A PRACTITIONER

In the United States, practitioners tend to focus on only one or two aspects of Chinese medicine like acupuncture or massage. And licensing varies from state to state. For example, doctors of oriental medicine (OMDs) are licensed in some states to prescribe herbal remedies and to perform acupuncture. Some Western practitioners have also incorporated aspects of Chinese medicine into their practices.

The following organization offers referrals of certified or licensed practitioners.

- The National Certification Commission for Acupuncture and Oriental Medicine
  (703) 548-9004
  www.nccaom.org

- The American Association of Oriental Medicine
  (866) 455-7999
  www.aaom.org

- American Academy of Acupuncture
  (323) 937-5514
  www.medicalacupuncture.org

Chiropractic

Common uses:

To treat back pain and other painful conditions.

Chiropractic is the manipulation of the spine to relieve pain and restore normal movement. Although it's been practiced since the late 18th century, conventional medicine questioned its usefulness for years. However, in 1987, a group of chiropractors sued the American Medical Association for restraint of trade. Since then chiropractic has been increasingly accepted as part of conventional care. The idea behind chiropractic is that malalignment of the vertebrae, which house the spinal cord, affects our entire system. Chiropractors work by manually adjusting any part of the spine that seems misaligned. Some chiropractors also use electrical stimulation, ultrasound, homeopathy, herbs and nutritional counseling.

SCIENTIFIC EVIDENCE

There is no evidence suggesting that chiropractic can treat the wide variety of ailments some practitioners claim. But a number of studies do suggest that chiropractic can be effective in relieving back pain. In a Canadian study of 30 patients with chronic back pain, those who received intensive chiropractic treatment had less pain and disability for a longer period than the control group. [J Manipulative Physiol Ther. 2004 Oct; 27 (8): 509-14.] A study of 72 patients with low back pain showed that those received chiropractic treatment four times a week experienced more relief than those treated only once a week. [Spine J. 2004 Sep-Oct; 4 (5): 574-83.] A randomized clinical trial showed that chiropractic was more helpful in reducing pain than placebo. [J Manipulative Physiol Ther. 2004 Jul-Aug; 27 (6) 388-98.]

SIDE EFFECTS AND INTERACTIONS

- Tell your chiropractor if you are taking anticoagulants. Chiropractic can increase bleeding or bruising.

SAFETY CONCERNS

- If you have arthritis or severe back pain, consult your doctor before trying chiropractic.

- Beware of practitioners who claim that chiropractic can fix anything such as bedwetting or infections.

- Do not let your chiropractor take repeat X-rays.

- Stop treatment if your symptoms get worse or if you see no improvement after a month.

FINDING A PRACTITIONER

Chiropractors are licensed in all states following four years of chiropractic training. Ask your doctor to refer you to someone or contact the following organization for information about finding a practitioner.

- American Chiropractic Association
  (800) 986-4636
  www.amerchiro.org

Chondroitin Sulfate

Common uses:

To strengthen and protect cartilage from breakdown.

Chondroitin sulfate is a natural component of cartilage that blocks enzymes destructive to cartilage tissue. It also helps cartilage retain water and elasticity. The supplement form comes from cattle trachea, shark cartilage, or in synthetic form, and it's been used in Europe for years as a treatment for osteoarthritis. Although it may help add stability to joints damaged by rheumatoid arthritis, it will not repair cartilage damage resulting from immune dysfunction and inflammation. It's often sold in combination with glucosamine, another compound involved in cartilage formation and repair.

SCIENTIFIC EVIDENCE

A number of studies suggest that chondroitin is better than placebo at relieving joint discomfort. It may not be more effective than NSAIDs but it has fewer negative side effects and longer lasting effects. A one-year, double-blind Swiss study found that patients with osteoarthritis taking chondroitin had less pain and improved knee function than those taking placebos. [Osteoarthritis Cartilage. 2004 Apr; 12 (4): 269-76.] A double-blind Australian study of osteoarthritis patients found that a topical application of glucosamine and chondroitin reduced knee pain within four weeks. [J Rheumatol. 2003 Mar; 30 (3): 523-8.] A Belgian meta-analysis of clinical trials between 1980 and 2002 also found that chondroitin was effective at relieving pain and increasing mobility. [Arch Intern Med. 2003 Jul 14; 163 (13): 1514-22.] The NIH is currently studying how chondroitin works in combination with glucosamine; the results of those studies are expected in 2005.

SIDE EFFECTS AND INTERACTIONS

- May cause nausea and indigestion.

- It may increase bleeding if you are taking drugs or herbs that are blood thinners.

SAFETY CONCERNS

- Do not take chondroitin derived from shark cartilage. It may have heavy metal contamination.

- Do not take if you are pregnant.

DOSAGE

1,200 mg a day. It's most commonly taken with gluco-somine, although no studies suggest that they are more effective together than alone.

CMO (cetyl myristoleate; cerasomal-cis-9-cetylmyristoleate)

Common uses:

To treat most forms of arthritis.

CMO's effectiveness and safety are unproven. CMO in supplement form comes from beef tallow.

SCIENTIFIC EVIDENCE

This supplement has been touted by some as a cure for arthritis since 1994 when a promising study at NIH concluded that rats injected with CMO were protected from arthritis. [J Pharm Sco. 1994 Mar; 83 (3): 296-9.) A 2003 study that injected rats with CMO also found a reduction in the incidence of arthritis and in the symptoms of those rats that did develop arthritis. Their findings were less dramatic, however, than those in the 1994 study. (Pharmacol Res. 2003 Jan; 47 (1): 43-7.) But research hasn't gone much beyond that – and there has been no published human research.

SIDE EFFECTS AND INTERACTIONS
- Corticosteroids and methotrexate may interfere with CMO.

SAFETY CONCERNS
- Do not stop taking your arthritis medications – corticosteroids or methotrexate – to take CMO. CMO has not been proven safe or effective.

DOSAGE
Take capsules as directed for 10 to 20 days.

Coconut Oil

Common uses:

To boost the immune system and support metabolic functions; to kill infectious organisms; promote healthy skin; ease digestion.

Coconut oil is a saturated tropical oil. It differs from other oils because it has what are called medium-chain triglycerides instead of long-chain ones. Its fats get into the bloodstream more quickly than other fats, making them an excellent and fast energy source. The fats also go directly to the liver so that little is converted to fat in the body. In supplement form, the oil used as an antimicrobial for conditions such as intestinal yeast infections.

SCIENTIFIC EVIDENCE

Some researchers believe that the capric and lauric acids in coconut oil can support the immune system by fighting microorganisms involved in conditions such as herpes simplex and HIV. A small clinical trial in the Philippines showed that 50 percent of HIV patients consuming coconut oil had a reduced viral count and increased number of immune cells. [Reprowatch. 1999 Feb 1-28:6,11.) Mice fed coconut oil for five weeks had lowered inflammatory responses than those fed olive or safflower oil, suggesting a possible anti-inflammatory property. [Immunology. 1999 Mar; 96(3): 404-10.] The research regarding coconut oil and heart disease is mixed. In a study of diets high in lauric acid (a large component of coconut oil), levels of LDL (bad) cholesterol and total cholesterol were significantly raised. [American J Clinical Nutrition 56 (5): 895-898 (Nov 1992)]. But in a 2004 study, rats fed coconut oil for 45 days had a reduction of total cholesterol, triglycerides and LDL, and an increase in HDL [Clin Biochem. 2004 Sep; 37 (9): 830-5.] Some studies have also shown that the medium-chain triglycerides in coconut oil speed up metabolism.

SIDE EFFECTS AND INTERACTIONS
• Eating high amounts of coconut oil on an empty stomach may cause stomach upset.

SAFETY CONCERNS
• May increase cholesterol and triglyceride blood levels.

DOSAGE

Four tablespoons a day (25 grams of lauric acid) are recommended to boost immunity.

Coenzyme Q-10

Common uses:

To help fight fibromyalgia, chronic fatigue and Parkinson's disease; to treat heart disease; to control high blood pressure; to prevent and treat cancer; to counter Alzheimer's and memory loss; to treat gum disease.

Coenzyme Q10 has been nicknamed vitamin Q because of its role in keeping the body running smoothly. It's found in every human cell – particularly in the heart – and in most foods. The Q stands for compounds called quinines that work with enzymes to produce chemical reactions throughout the body, particularly reactions that support the heart muscles. In fact people with heart disease tend to lack coenzyme Q10. Co Q10 is also a powerful anti-oxidant that prevents cellular damage by unstable oxygen molecules called free radicals.

SCIENTIFIC EVIDENCE

Studies indicate the Co Q10 in combination with prescription medications can be effective in treating congestive heart failure. For example, ten out of 13 double-blind studies have drawn that conclusion. [Biofactors. 2003; 18 (1-4): 79-89.] Studies on its effect on fibromyalgia have been mixed. Some researchers believe that a deficiency of Co Q10 could lead to a lack of adenosine triphosphate (ATP), a molecule believed to be lacking in those with fibromyalgia. But a 1998 study found no difference in the level of Co Q10 in those with fibromyalgia and in healthy people. [Clin Exp Rheumatol 1998; 16: 513] In an open, controlled study of patients with fibromyalgia, however, 64 percent of those given 200 mg of Co Q10 and 200 mg of ginkgo biloba extract felt significantly better after 84 days than they did at the outset. [J Int Med Res. 2002 Mar-Apr.; 30 (2): 195-9.]

SIDE EFFECTS AND INTERACTIONS

- May experience stomach upset or nausea, headache, difficulty sleeping or flu-like symptoms.

- If you take anticoagulants (prescription drugs or supplements), do not take coenzyme Q10 without consulting your doctor. It may increase the risk of bleeding.

- May increase the risk of blood clots.

- Vitamin E may augment the effects of coenzyme Q10.

SAFETY CONCERNS

- Pregnant and nursing women and those with heart disease should check with their doctor before taking coenzyme Q10.

DOSAGE

There is no established dose, although a typical dose is 50 mg twice a day.

Collagen

Common uses:
To treat rheumatoid and juvenile rheumatoid arthritis.

Collagen is a substance extracted from animal cartilage. One type, type II collagen, appears to suppress the autoimmune response that attacks healthy joints in those with rheumatoid arthritis.

SCIENTIFIC EVIDENCE

Studies of type II collagen have been mixed. In an Italian double-blind study of 60 patients with rheumatoid arthritis who were treated with type II collagen for six months, the patients showed only small and inconsistent benefits. [Clin Exp Rehummatol. 2000 Sep-Oct; 18 (5): 571-7.] In a randomized controlled trial of 190 patients with rheumatoid arthritis, those patients taking type II collagen showed no improvement. [Arthritis Rheum. 1999 June; 42 (6): 1204-8.] However, other studies have been more positive. A Harvard University double-blind study of 60 people with rheumatoid arthritis found that those who took type II collagen for three months had significant improvement in swollen, tender joints than did those taking a placebo. {Science September 24 1993] In a multi-center, double blind study of 275 patients with rheumatoid arthritis, significant improvements were seen even at the lowest of four doses given over 24 weeks when compared to placebo. [Arthritis Rheum. 1998 Feb; 41 (2): 290-7.]

SIDE EFFECTS AND INTERACTIONS

• May cause nausea.

SAFETY CONCERNS

• Taking animal cartilage is not the same as taking Type II collagen.

• Make sure that the collagen product you take does not contain herbs or other supplements.

DOSAGE

500 micrograms or less a day.

Colostrum

Common uses:

To improve muscle endurance and boost tissue repair; control diarrhea in those with immune deficiencies; help minimize stomach upset caused by NSAIDs.

Colostrum is the first milk from a cow following the birth of a calf. It is rich in growth factors (which stimulate cell and tissue growth), antibodies, vitamins, minerals and high-quality protein.

SCIENTIFIC EVIDENCE

A double-blind study found significant improvement in exercise performance in athletes taking bovine colostrum over eight weeks compared to the placebo group. [Int J Sport Nutr Exerc Metab 2002; 12: 461-469.] Another double-blind study found that elite rowers who took colostrum had a significantly stronger athletic performance than those taking a placebo. [Int J Sport Nutr Exerc Metab 2002; 12: 349-365.] Studies of colostrum's effect in preventing stomach distress sometimes brought on by NSAIDs indicated that it's helpful in those who take NSAIDs intermittently, not chronically. [Clin Sci (Lond) 2001; 100: 627-633.] A number of studies suggest that colostrum is helpful in curbing diarrhea in those with immune deficiencies. In a double-blind trial, 80 children with diarrhea due to a viral infection received collostrum or placebo. By day four, 33 of those receiving collostrum were diarrhea-free compared to only 21 in the placebo group. And 95 percent of those taking collostrum were free of the virus versus only 50 percent of those taking placebo. [Acta Paediatr 1995; 84: 996-1001.]

SIDE EFFECTS AND INTERACTIONS

- Do not use if you are allergic to cow's milk.

- Children may experience flu-like symptoms.

- May cause gas and nausea.

SAFETY CONCERNS

- You should only purchase fresh colostrum from someone licensed by the USDA.

DOSAGE

10 to 60 grams per day is the range found helpful in various studies.

Comfrey Root

Common uses:

Used externally to heal superficial wounds, reduce inflammation and pain in conditions like arthritis. Taken internally to soothe coughs, ulcers, hernias, colitis, and to stop internal bleeding or diarrhea; to loosen congestion; to treat mouth sores and bleeding gums.

Comfrey is an herb found in moist meadows or along river banks, where it may grow four feet tall. Its root has been used medically for more than 2,000 years to speed healing both inside and out. A compound called allantoin is thought to be the primary healer within comfrey root. But comfrey also contains vitamins A and B12, as well as calcium, potassium and phosphorus.

SCIENTIFIC EVIDENCE

Comfrey is dangerous when used internally. However, a number of studies attest to comfrey's healing effect when used topically. In double-blind study of 142 patients suffering from ankle sprains, pain was reduced by 63 percent after 8 days in those who applied comfrey ointment four times a day. That was true for only 25 percent of those treated with placebo. Swelling was reduced by 61 percent (versus 36 percent for placebo). [Phytotherapie 2000; 21: 127-134.] In a placebo-controlled study of 41 patients with musculoskeletal inflammatory conditions, patients treated with comfrey ointment felt some relief compared to placebo. [Planta Medica 1993; 59: A703.] In a multi-center German study, more than two thirds of patients with painful conditions were able to reduce or stop taking anti-inflammatory drugs. [Fortschr Med Orig. 2002; 120 (1): 1-9.]

SIDE EFFECTS AND INTERACTIONS

- No known side effects of external applications. Internal use may damage the liver.

SAFETY CONCERNS

- Should not be used externally by pregnant women or nursing mothers, or internally by anyone.

- Contains alkaloids that are harmful to the liver and may be cancer causing, even in small amounts.

- Do not use on deep wounds since it may heal the surface before the deeper wound.

- Do not use for more than four weeks.

DOSAGE

Comes in ointments, salves and oil extract for external treatment. Do not use more than four weeks.

Copper

Common uses:

Helps bone growth and may prevent bone loss; as an anti-inflammatory.

Copper is an essential trace metal found in nuts, chocolate, seeds and dried beans. It helps bone growth and may prevent bone loss. It's also necessary for the production of connective tissue, which is damaged in rheumatoid arthritis. Certain conditions like osteoporosis and bone abnormalities are associated with copper deficiencies. Copper is also an anti-inflammatory and may boost the effectiveness of NSAIDs. As an anti-oxidant, it helps protect cells from free radicals as well.

SCIENTIFIC EVIDENCE

A review of uncontrolled studies from 1940 to 1971 involving 1,500 patients with different forms of arthritis showed that copper helped some people with rheumatoid arthritis, ankylosing spondylitis, gout and Reiter's syndrome. The studies aren't conclusive but it's worth making sure you get at least 3 mg, including what you get from food sources. A University of California study showed that calcium and vitamin D are more effective at increasing bone density and preventing osteoporosis when used in combination with copper, zinc and manganese. [J Nutr. 1994 Jul; 124 (7): 1060-4] Otherwise, the research is scant regarding copper and arthritis.

SIDE EFFECTS AND INTERACTIONS
• May cause nausea, vomiting, diarrhea or anemia.

SAFETY CONCERNS

- People with Wilson's disease – a disorder that causes copper to accumulate in the body – should never take copper.

- Exceeding the daily requirement is dangerous and may cause nausea, vomiting, stomach pain, diarrhea, dizziness, headache and a metallic taste in your mouth.

DOSAGE

2 to 3 mgs per day of copper chelate. As much as 2 grams are found in many multivitamins. If you have copper plumbing you are also getting copper in your drinking water. And as indicated above, copper is in a number of common foods. So a supplement may create an overdose.

Copper Bracelets

Common uses:
To reduce joint pain of arthritis.

Wearing copper bracelets to reduce rheumatic pain is an old folk remedy that little, if any, science bears out.

SCIENTIFIC EVIDENCE

If someone lacks copper, it's possible that the copper in a copper bracelet may be absorbed through the skin, making up for the deficiency. But there's very little science to suggest this is an effective remedy for arthritis.

SIDE EFFECTS AND INTERACTIONS

None

SAFETY CONCERNS

None

DOSAGE

Humans need 2-3 mg a day of copper. Chances are you won't be getting that from a bracelet. More effective sources are foods such as nuts, chocolate, seeds and dried beans, or taking a supplement.

Coral Calcium

Common uses:

Treatment for lupus, multiple sclerosis, cancer, fatigue, gallstones, indigestion and heart disease.

Coral calcium is mined from coral reefs off the coast of Okinawa, Japan. The reef has a shell composed of calcium carbonate, magnesium, and trace minerals. The calcium does not cure disease. In fact both the FDA and FTC have asked those marketing coral calcium to eliminate the false advertising.

SCIENTIFIC EVIDENCE

Calcium regulates nerve and muscle function, builds bones, and may prevent colon cancer, kidney stones, periodontal disease and high blood pressure. But there is no evidence that it can cure diseases like lupus, multiple sclerosis and heart disease.

SIDE EFFECTS AND INTERACTIONS
None

SAFETY CONCERNS
- Calcium carbonate supplements are safer and far less expensive than coral calcium.
- Some calcium supplements contain lead. Make sure the label says lead free.

DOSAGE
1,000 to 1,500 mg daily for women; 700 mg for men. It's preferable to get most of that from food.

Cranberry Seed Oil

Common uses:

To keep body cells healthy, particularly skin cells.

Cranberry seed oil is pressed from the seeds of American cranberries. Its power lies in its blend of omega- 3, -6 and -9 essential fatty acids that are essential to skin, heart, brain and total health of the cells. It has an advantage over fish and flax oil, both of which also contain essential fatty acids: unlike those, it contains anti-oxidants that can keep it fresh for two years.

SCIENTIFIC EVIDENCE

Although there has been little research on cranberry seed oil, a number of positive studies have been on fatty acids. In a review of studies done between 1979 and 1995, researchers found that treatment with omega-3 fatty acids was more effective in treating rheumatoid arthritis than placebo. [Semin Arthritis Rheum. 1998 Jun;27(6):366-70.] Reseachers in Spain noted that RA patients have a deficiency in fatty acids, which may explain why fatty acid supplement appear to be beneficial. [Jrl Rheum, Vol.25, Feb 2000, p 298-303.]In a double-blind, placebo-controlled study, those with RA took omega-3 and -6 fatty acids for four months. However, the researchers saw no benefit compared to placebo and concluded they need more information about effective doses. [Eur J Clin Nutr. 2004 Jun;58(6):839-45.] A earlier review of studies and case reports concluded that omega-3 and omega-6 fatty acids do have an anti-inflammatory effect but do not correct the immune system dysfunction in RA. [Hawaii Med J. 1999 May; 58 (5): 126-31.]

SIDE EFFECTS AND INTERACTIONS

None

SAFETY CONCERNS

None

DOSAGE

As directed.

Craniosacral Therapy

Common uses:

To ease pain, particularly headaches, and to promote relaxation.

The therapy involves gentle manipulation of the skull, spine, and pelvis (the craniosacral system) to ease the flow of fluids within the system. Its practitioners believe that the movement of fluids creates an essential body rhythm that affects health, especially when blocked. No studies prove the therapy's effectiveness although patients do report relief. William Garner Sutherland, an American osteopath began the method in the 1930s based on his belief that the bones of the skull were designed for movement. Sessions last from 20 minutes to an hour.

SCIENTIFIC EVIDENCE

No clinical trials prove that this method works. However, anecdotal evidence suggests it can relieve headache pain, sinusitis and reduce stress.

SIDE EFFECTS AND INTERACTIONS

None

SAFETY CONCERNS

- Be sure to see a qualified therapist, particularly if applying this therapy to an infant.

- If you have had a brain hemorrhage or aneurysm, check with your doctor before using this therapy.

FINDING A PRACTITIONER

Practitioners are usually physical or massage therapists or chiropractors as well. Look for someone who has special training in the method. You can also contact The Upledger Institute, Inc. for referrals of trained therapists. (800) 233-5880. www.upledger.com.

Creatine

Common uses:

To increase muscle energy; to relieve muscle pain from sports activity.

Creatine is a substance naturally produced by the liver. It's also available in protein foods like meats and fish. Creatine helps muscles produce adenosine triphosphate (ATP), which fuels cell energy. It's often used in supplement form by athletes to enhance performance. However, some athletes get no benefit from creatine.

SCIENTIFIC EVIDENCE

In a study of twelve patients with rheumatoid arthritis, eight of those treated with creatine for three weeks showed an increase of muscle strength. But disease activity remained the same and function didn't improve either. [Rheumatology (Oxford). 2000 Mar; 39 (3): 293-8] A double-blind study of 36 patients with muscular dystrophies found that significant improvement in strength and daily activities in those who took creatine as opposed to those who took the placebo. [Neurology 2000 May 9; 54 (9): 1848-50.] In two clinical trials of patients with a neuromuscular disease, patients showed a significant increase in strength after treatment.

SIDE EFFECTS AND INTERACTIONS

• Can cause dehydration, stomach cramps and diarrhea.

• Can cause water retention if taken at higher than recommended doses.

SAFETY CONCERNS

• Stick to recommended dosages. Excess amounts may be harmful to the liver and kidneys. Besides, the body can use only so much creatine; the rest is eliminated as waste.

• Do not take immediately before or during exercise.

• Do not take if you are exercising outdoors in the heat. It can lead to dehydration.

• Long-term use can damage the kidneys.

• Do not take high doses if you are already taking NSAIDs because of the added stress on the kidneys.

DOSAGE

• Buy creatine monohydrate, the form used in most clinical studies.

• For exercise performance, take 2-4 teaspoons mixed with juice for five days, then only one teaspoon per day.

• For muscle aches, pains and sports-related injuries, takes one teaspoon twice a day mixed with juice until you no longer feel a benefit.

D-f

Deep Tissue Massage

Common uses:

To relieve chronic tension and low-back pain; relax tight muscles that surround arthritic joints; break up scar tissue.

Deep tissue massages is the application of strong pressure on deep muscle or tissue layers to relieve tension. The practitioner often strokes across the grain of the muscles using his fingers, thumbs and even his elbows. This can result in soreness, especially in preliminary sessions. When muscles are stressed, they block oxygen and nutrients, which can lead to inflammation and a buildup of toxins in the tissue. Deep tissue massage helps loosen the muscle tissues, releasing the toxins, and allowing blood and oxygen flow.

SCIENTIFIC EVIDENCE

- See "Massage," p. 159.

SIDE EFFECTS AND INTERACTIONS

- You may experience some soreness, especially after the first few sessions.

SAFETY CONCERNS

None

FINDING A PRACTITIONER

See "Massage," p. 159.

Devil's Claw

Common uses:
To relieve pain, digestive problems, inflammation.

The many small hooks that cover the plant's fruit also supply its name. The root of the African plant contains a painkilling and anti-inflammatory chemical called harpagoside. Although it's been touted as a remedy for a number of conditions, it's most effective as a pain reliever.

SCIENTIFIC EVIDENCE
Studies are mixed. In a French study, those with arthritis pain took devil's claw for three weeks with no significant relief of inflammation. [Prostaglandins Leukot Essent Fatty Acids. 1992 Aug; 46 (4): 283-6.] In a multi-center German study of patients with osteoarthritis of the hip or knee, patients treated with devil's claw showed continuous improvement in pain over the twelve-week study. [Phytother Res. 2003 Dec.; 17 (10): 1165-72.] And in a Canadian review of studies, authors concluded that the use of 60 mg or more daily of devil's claw was effective in treating pain. [BMC Complement Altern Med. 2004 Sep 15; 4(1): 13.]

SIDE EFFECTS AND INTERACTIONS
- May cause diarrhea and upset stomach.
- May increase stomach acid. Do not use if you have ulcers.

- Do not take with antacids, H2 antagonists such as cimetidine (*Tagamet*), famotidine (*Pepcid*) and ranitidine (*Zantac*), or proton pump inhibitors such as lansoprazole (*Prevacid*) and omeprazole (*Prilosec*).

- May decrease blood sugar levels. If you are being treated for diabetes, consult your doctor before using devil's claw.

- May increase the risk of bleeding when used with anticoagulants, NSAIDs, or blood-thinning herbs, such as ginkgo biloba and garlic.

SAFETY CONCERNS

- Do not use if you are pregnant or nursing. Devil's claw may stimulate contractions.

DOSAGE

50 to 100 mg of standardized harpagoside taken on an empty stomach.

DHEA

Common uses:

To treat Addison's disease, menopause, lupus, rheumatoid arthritis, fatigue

DHEA is a male hormone made by the adrenal glands and converted into testosterone and estrogen. Both men and women produce DHEA, and its levels drop with age. DHEA levels are low in those with rheumatoid arthritis and juvenile rheumatoid arthritis. At 60, we make only 15 percent the amount we did at 20. For that reason, in part, it has been marketed as a supplement that tackles age-related problems such as osteoporosis, cancer, weight gain and lowered sex drive. Science doesn't support most of the claims. However, DHEA does appear effective in treating lupus, Addison's disease (adrenal insufficiency) and some menopausal symptoms.

SCIENTIFIC EVIDENCE

Studies on DHEA are mixed. When 280 healthy men and women over 60 took DHEA for one year in a French double-blind study, there was no change in muscle function and strength. [Arch Intern Med. 2003 Mar 24; 163 (6): 720-7.] A recent study showed DHEA is beneficial for women with lupus (SLE). [Arthritis Rheum. 2002; 46:2924-7.] However, in a German study on mice with induced arthritis taking DHEA, the DHEA did lessen the synptom severity. [Inflamm Res. 2004 May; 53 (5): 189-98. Epub 2004 Apr 21.] In an Italian study, rats given DHEA had immune responses restored that had been weakened by age. [J Immunol. 2002 Feb 15; 168 (4): 1753-8.]

SIDE EFFECTS AND INTERACTIONS

- May cause headache, fatigue, nasal congestion.
- Large doses may cause women to develop acne, facial hair, deepening voice, mood swings; men on large doses

may experience higher blood pressure, aggression or breast tenderness.

- May raise blood sugar levels. If you have diabetes, check with your doctor before taking DHEA.

- May change the way the liver breaks down some drugs, such as triazolam (*Halcion*), raising the levels of the drugs. Taking DHEA with azathioprine (*Imuran*) or methotrexate may damage the liver.

- Drugs such as alprazolamm (*Xanax*) may increase DHEA levels, which in turn could raise side effects.

- May reduce levels of HDL, the good cholesterol.

SAFETY CONCERNS

- Take DHEA only under a doctor's supervision and only after he has determined that your DHEA level is low.

- In theory, may heighten the risk of breast, ovarian or prostrate cancer. Ask your doctor to examine you for any hormone-related cancers before you take DHEA.

- Women who are pregnant or nursing should not take this supplement.

- May raise the risk of blood clots.

- DHEA is a manufactured chemical, stronger than many herbs or nutrients. Its long-term safety is unknown.

DOSAGE

No more than 25 mg a day for men. As little as 5 to 10 mg a week can maintain normal levels of DHEA in the blood. In an ongoing study, women are taking 200 mg per day, but your doctor would likely start you on something much lower.

DMSO

Common uses:

To relieve joint and soft tissue inflammation; to treat interstitial cystitis, a bladder condition; to protect organs during transplants; to protect frozen human tissue (embryos, stem cells, bone marrow).

DMSO, a by-product of wood processing, is a chemical used in paint thinner and antifreeze. But it's also used for medical purposes, taken both externally and internally. In the 1960s, it received a lot of attention as a therapy for many kinds of arthritis. However in animal studies during the mid-60s, very high doses of DMSO damaged the animals' eye lens. This has not been true in human studies. Since then it's been approved by the FDA only to treat interstitial cystitis.

SCIENTIFIC EVIDENCE

Despite its controversy, many DMSO studies on humans have been positive. In a German double-blind study, 112 patients with osteoarthritis of the knee, DMSO applied over three weeks was an effective pain reliever compared to placebo. [Fortschr Med. 1995 Nov 10; 113 (31): 446-50.] In a Swedish double-blind study of 150 patients with some kind of tendon-related pain,

44 percent of the patients were pain-free after 14 days of DMSO topical treatment compared to only 9 percent of the placebo group. [Fortschr Med. 1994 Apr 10; 112 (10): 142-6.] In an Irish study of 23 patients treated for interstitial cystitis with DMSO, 17 responded well to treatment. [Cathy McLean, Dept. of Urology, Gartnavel General Hospital, Glasgow, Scotland, 2000].

SIDE EFFECTS AND INTERACTIONS

- May cause bad breath or a taste like garlic and onions.

- May cause an allergic reaction, or skin irritation and itching.

- Do not take with other blood-thinning agents.

- May cause headache, nausea or rash.

SAFETY CONCERNS

- Do not buy DMSO yourself. If it is not pure, it can be dangerous, causing skin irritation; kidney, liver and vision problems; and speed up joint deterioration.

DOSAGE

DMSO is used orally, intravenously, through injection, applied topically. Used topically, apply doses of 60 to 90 percent DMSO one to three times a day.

FINDING A PRACTITIONER

Ask a doctor to help you find and use DMSO appropriately. You can also contact Oregon Health Sciences

University in Portland, Oregon, which has a program for treatment: www.oshuhealth.com

Echinacea

Common uses:

Fights colds, flu and other infections.

Echinacea is a native North American wildflower used to boost the immune system. It's approved in Germany by the national health agency for upper respiratory infections, wounds and lower urinary tract infections. The research in the United States has been inconclusive. It is not known how it affects those with already overactive immune systems; experts advise those with arthritis and other auto-immune conditions not to take it.

SCIENTIFIC EVIDENCE

Study results have been mixed. In a Canadian double-blind study of 128 people with a cold, those who took echinacea had 23.1 percent less severe cold symptoms than those in the placebo group. [J Clin Pharm Ther. 2004 Feb; 29 (1): 75-83.] But in a Seattle study, children with upper respiratory tract infections did not respond to treatment with echinacea and had an increased risk of rash. [JAMA 2003 Dec 3; 290 (21): 2824-30.] A 2000 review of studies to date concluded that echinacea is effective not for prevention but for reducing the duration and severity of upper respiratory infections. [Biochem Phrmacol. 2000 Jul 15; 60(2): 155-8.] A 2003 review drew similar conclusions. [Integr Cancer Ther. 2003 Sep; 2 (3): 247-67.]

SIDE EFFECTS AND INTERACTIONS

- May interact with conventional drugs.

- Do not take with corticosteroids or other immunosuppressive drugs.

SAFETY CONCERNS

- Should not be taken by those with autoimmune conditions like rheumatoid arthritis.

- Do not take with drugs like methotrexate that affect the liver. It may contribute to liver damage.

DOSAGE

Limit use to eight weeks. Follow dosage recommended by the manufacturer.

Feldenkrais Method

Common uses:

To improve posture and reduce muscle tension.

The Feldenkrais method is an education technique on how to move and stand in ways that can relieve physical tension and stress. Such relief allows a greater range of motion and flexibility. The method is often recommended by doctors and physical therapists because the movements are so gentle. It's an ideal method for those with arthritis to learn before taking up more strenuous activity since it teaches them how to move in a way that will help protect them from injury. The method is taught one on one or in classes.

SCIENTIFIC EVIDENCE

Studies have revolved around four areas: pain management; functional performance and motor control; psychological effects, and quality of life. In a Swedish study comparing three physical therapy approaches for patients with musculoskeletal disorders, researchers found that Feldenkrais and body awareness therapy improved quality of life and control of pain. [Disabil Rehavil. 2002 Apr 15; 24 (6): 308-17.] A study of 34 chronic pain patients using Feldenkrais showed reduced pain, improved function, with continued independent use of the therapy two years after discharge. [Presented at CSM in Boston in Feb. 1998.] A very small study of five fibromyalgia patients showed increased management of daily living activities as the result of Feldenkrais training. [Presented at the Feldenkrais Guild Conference in Aug., 1997.]

SIDE EFFECTS AND INTERACTIONS

None

SAFETY CONCERNS

None

FINDING A PRACTITIONER

To be certified, Feldenkrais practitioners much have 800-1,000 hours of training in three to four years. Ask your doctor or physical therapist to refer you to a certified practitioner. Or you can contact the Feldenkrais Guild of North America, (800) 775-2118; www.feldenkrais.com

Fish Oil

Common uses:

To reduce inflammation and pain, especially in rheumatoid arthritis; to help maintain a healthy nervous system, cell walls and vision; improve Raynaud's phenomenon; to improve heart health; to help prevent some cancers

A number of studies show that oil from cold water fish such as salmon and mackerel help reduce inflammation and pain from rheumatoid arthritis. It's the omega-3 fatty acids that do the work, providing the building blocks for anti-inflammatory agents. The acids also help preserve a healthy nervous system, cell walls and vision. And they improve heart health by thinning the blood and lowering triglycerides. In fact, the American Heart Association recommends that those with no history of heart disease eat fish twice a week, and daily for those with heart disease. Fish oil may also prevent some cancers.

SCIENTIFIC EVIDENCE

At least 13 randomized, controlled trials have demonstrated that fish oil does have beneficial, anti-inflammatory effects on those with rheumatoid arthritis. {Drugs. 2003; 63 (9): 845-53.] A major review of inflammatory diseases and diet points out that fish oils can significantly reduce morning stiffness and painful joints in rheumatoid arthritis patients. [British Journal of Nutrition, Vol. 85, March 2001, pp. 251-69.] An Australian 15-week study of 50 patients with rheumatoid arthritis found major improvements in those receiving fish oil, particularly in morning stiffness and overall disease activity. [Journal of Rheumatology, Vol. 27, October 2000, pp 2343-46.] An accompanying editorial about the study suggested that fish oil now become part of standard therapy for rheumatoid arthritis patients. [Journal of Rheumatology, Vol. 27, October 2000,pp. 2305-06]

SIDE EFFECTS AND INTERACTIONS

• May intensify the effect of blood-thinning drugs, or herbs like garlic and turmeric.

SAFETY CONCERNS

• Be careful if you take cod liver oil. You may get too much vitamin A and D.

DOSAGE

3,000 mg of the fish oil components eicosapentaenoic acid (EPA) and docosahexaenoic acid (DHA) a day.

Flaxseed

Common uses:

To reduce inflammation in rheumatoid arthritis; to ease symptoms in Raynaud's phenomenon; to boost heart health; to prevent some cancers.

Flaxseeds provide an essential fatty acid called alpha-linolenic acid (ALA), which is converted by the body into the same omega-3 fatty acids found in some fish. Omega-3 fatty acids help fight inflammation and lower heart disease risk by lowering blood pressure and cholesterol. Flaxseeds also contain a particular phytoestrogen, or plant estrogen, called lignans that may help prevent breast cancer. In fact, in mice studies, offspring of mothers fed flaxseed had lowered risk of breast cancer compared to the control group. Flaxseed may also reduce menopausal symptoms like hot flashes.

SCIENTIFIC EVIDENCE

In a Finnish study of 22 patients with rheumatoid arthritis, flaxseed oil had no benefit. [Rheumatol Int. 1995; 14(6): 231-4.] A review of studies and case reports concluded that omega-3 and omega-6 fatty acids do have an anti-inflammatory effect but does not correct the immune system dysfunction in RA. [Hawaii Med J. 1999 May; 58 (5): 126-31.] And the data regarding flaxseed's contribution to heart health looks good but not yet solid. Human studies show that flaxseed lowers cholesterol and decreases inflammation but whether it lowers blood pressure or helps prevent clogged arteries is not clear. [Nutr Rev. 2004 Jan; 62 (1): 18-27.] A number of Canadian animal studies show that flaxseed may prevent breast cancer or block its spread but few human studies have confirmed that. In a small study, the tumor growth in women who ate flaxseed daily slowed compared to the control group. [Goss, 2001]

SIDE EFFECTS AND INTERACTIONS

- You may experience some gas and loose bowels when you first start eating flaxseed. Start with small amounts and work up to the recommended daily amount.

SAFETY CONCERNS

None

DOSAGE

One fourth of a cup of ground flaxseed or 1-3 table-spoons of flaxseed oil a day. However, many of the cancer-preventive lignans are processed out of the oil. Do not use capsules, which are even more processed than the oil.

G-j

Gamma Linoleic Acid

 (GLA; evening primrose oil and borage oil)

Common uses:

To relieve pain and inflammation of rheumatoid arthritis.

The body produces GLA from linoleic acid, an essential fatty acid obtained from corn, sunflower, soy and peanut oils. The body converts GLA into prostaglandins, which fight inflammation and help regulate blood pressure and other body processes. GLA may help quell the inflammation of arthritis and may benefit those with lupus. One study indicated that it may be helpful in boosting the effect of the breast-cancer drug, tamoxifen. And combined with fish oil, it may boost the benefits of calcium in strengthening bones and preventing osteoporosis.

SCIENTIFIC EVIDENCE

A small number of studies suggest that GLA is effective treatment for those with rheumatoid arthritis. [Semin Arthritis Rheum. 1995 Oct; 25 (2): 87-96.] [Br J Nutr. 2001 Mar; 85 (3): 251-69.] A double-blind study of 56 patients with rheumatoid arthritis found that GLA was effective. [Arthrtis Rheum. 1996 Nov; 39 (11): 1808-17.] More recent studies, however, have been less promising. A double-blind study of rheumatoid arthritis patients in the Netherlands found no benefit from treatment with GLA over four months. [Eur J Clin Nutr. 2004 Jun; 58 (6): 839-45.] A Swedish double blind study also found no effect on patients with Sjögren's syndrome. [Scand J Rheumatol. 2002; 31 (2): 72-9.]

SIDE EFFECTS AND INTERACTIONS

- May augment the effect of prescription or herbal blood thinners.
- May cause nausea, diarrhea and stomach upset.
- May make epilepsy or seizures worsen.

SAFETY CONCERNS

None

DOSAGE

- 240 mg daily
- It may take six months before you will feel any effect from GLA.
- Take with food to enhance absorption.

Ginger

Common uses:
To relieve nausea, joint and muscle pain.

Most of us think of ginger as the tang in our cookies but it's also an herb that has been used for centuries in Chinese and Ayurvedic medicine to settle upset stomachs. It is an anti-oxidant and anti-inflammatory as well. It's thought to reduce pain by inhibiting the production of prostaglandins and leukotrienes, implicated in pain and swelling.

SCIENTIFIC EVIDENCE

A number of studies show ginger does relieve some pain in those with arthritis. In a six-week, double-blind study of 247 osteoarthritis patients given ginger extract, the ginger did reduce knee pain although there were some patients who got upset stomachs as well. [Arthritis Rheum. 2001 Nov.; 44 (11): 2461-2.] In a randomized controlled trial of 29 patients with osteoarthritis, the treatment group had less pain and handicap compared to the placebo group after six months. [Osteoarthritis Cartilage. 2003 Nov; 11 (11): 783-9.] A 2000 study had mixed results. In a cross-over study divided into three treatment periods of three weeks each (each followed by a week without treatment), researchers generally found no difference between placebo and ginger extract. However, in the first 3-week treatment period, ginger relieved pain better than placebo. [Osteoarthritis Cartilage. 2000 Jan; 8(1): 9-12.]

SIDE EFFECTS AND INTERACTIONS

- May cause occasional heartburn. Large doses may irritate stomach lining.

- May augment the risk of bleeding if taken with anticoagulant drugs or herbs.

- May increase the drowsiness of drugs such as lorazepam (*Ativan*), barbiturates (phenobarbital, narcotics, alcohol), and herbs such as valerian.

- May lower blood sugar levels. Anyone taking insulin should consult his doctor before taking ginger.

SAFETY CONCERNS

- Pregnant and nursing mothers should not take ginger without consulting their doctor.

- Do not use before surgery because of the risk of increased bleeding.

DOSAGE

One to four grams per day of fresh powdered ginger or 100-200 mg in pill form. But fresh or freeze-dried ginger may be more effective. A ¼ or ½ inch slice of ginger root is equivalent to a common dose. Drink it steeped in water or add to food.

Ginkgo (Ginkgo biloba)

Common uses:

To treat Alzheimer's disease, dementia, "fibro fog," or age-related memory loss; cerebral vascular disease, depression, Raynaud's phenomenon; poor circulation.

Chinese medicine has used the herb that comes from the leaves of ginkgo biloba trees for thousands of years. Ginkgo increases the blood flow to the brain and central nervous system and may also act as an anti-oxidant. It's thought to improve any number of conditions including memory difficulties, depression, impotence and asthma.

SCIENTIFIC EVIDENCE

The bulk of studies on ginkgo focus on memory. And a number of studies suggest that ginkgo can be helpful, particularly in Alzheimer's disease and dementia. [Curr Pharm Des. 2004; 10 (3): 261-4] [Pharmacopsychiatry. 2004 Nov; 36: 297-303.] But all studies aren't positive. In a 24-week Dutch study, those with dementia were no different after taking ginkgo than those in the placebo group. [J Clin Epidemiol. 2003 Apr; 56 (4): 367-76.]

SIDE EFFECTS AND INTERACTIONS

- May increase the risk of bleeding if taking with other anticoagulants.

- May cause upset stomach or headache.

- May increase blood pressure when combined with thiazide diuretics.

- Do not combine with insulin. Ginkgo may affect blood sugar levels.

SAFETY CONCERNS

- Ginkgo seeds and unprocessed ginkgo leaves are toxic. Do not use them.

- Do not take if you are pregnant or nursing.

- Do not combine with trazodone, an antidepressant, or with prochlorperazine, an antipsychotic drug.

- More than 240 mg a day may cause intoxication or disorientation.

DOSAGE

120-160 mg per day of standardized extracts containing 24 percent flavone glycosides (substances that act as anti-oxidants) and 6 percent terpene lactones (chemicals that improve blood flow). It may take six to nine weeks to notice an effect.

Ginseng

Common uses:

To treat fatigue, stress, diabetes, high blood pressure, impotence and male infertility; to improve cognitive function; to protect the liver.

There's no evidence to suggest that ginseng can help arthritis but it may boost energy. There are several types of ginseng: Asian (Panax ginseng), American (Panax quinquefolius) and Siberian (Eleutherococcus). Asian ginseng is the one most commonly used in supplements. Siberian ginseng has not been well studied. The root is the part of the plant used for medicine.

SCIENTIFIC EVIDENCE

Studies show some immune-strengthening activity. [Integr Cancer Ther. 2003 Sep; 2 (3): 247-67.] And research has indicated that Asian ginseng inhibits cancerous tumors. [Altern Med Rev. 2004 Sep; 9 (3): 259-74.] Ginseng may improve mood and cognitive performance as well. In a British study of healthy young adults, those taking ginseng showed improved memory compared to placebo.

SIDE EFFECTS AND INTERACTIONS

• May experience nervousness, stomach upset, insomnia or headaches. Caffeine can increase these effects.

• High doses of ginseng may affect menstruation and cause breast tenderness.

• Do not take with other anti-coagulants. May increase bleeding.

• May affect how other drugs or herbs react in the body, either increasing or decreasing their effect.

• May lower blood sugar levels. If you have diabetes, check with your doctor.

SAFETY CONCERNS

• Do not take if you are pregnant or nursing.

DOSAGE

The dosage depends on the amount of ginsenoside, the active ingredient. Look for supplements that have 7 percent ginsenoside. In pills and capsules, take 100 mg twice a day. Of the powdered root, take 500-1,000 mg a day. Stop taking for a week every two to three weeks.

Gin-Soaked Raisins

Common uses:
To ease arthritis aches.

Some people swear by this folk remedy. And it's true that the gin may temporarily dull pain and raisins do have anti-inflammatory effects. But you'd have to eat more than a handful to feel any relief.

SCIENTIFIC EVIDENCE
None

SAFETY CONCERNS

• Excess alcohol can make your symptoms worse by robbing your body of nutrients and contributing to depression.

DOSAGE
Skip the gin and eat some raisins as a snack or on your cereal.

Glucosamine

Common uses:
To ease osteoarthritis pain.

Glucosamine is a natural substance that supplies the building blocks to make and repair cartilage. Although there is no evidence that glucosamine supplements repair cartilage, studies suggest they can help relieve pain from osteoarthritis. The supplement is extracted from shellfish and taken in capsules. It takes several months to see any effect.

SCIENTIFIC EVIDENCE

In studies so far, glucosamine has shown just a small effect on osteoarthritis pain – and in some studies no effect at all. However, The National Center for Complementary and Alternative Medicine and the National Institute of Arthritis and Musculoskeletal and Skin Diseases (NIAMS) have funded the Glucosamine Arthritis Intervention Trial, a multi-centered placebo-controlled study, which expects to conclude in March 2005.[Med Health R I. 2004 Jun; 87(6): 176-9.] A double-blind study at Tufts New England Medical Center found glucosamine no more effective than placebo in relieving symptoms of knee osteoarthritis. [Am J Med. 2004 Nov 1; 117 ((): 643-9.] Similar results were reported by the Arthritis Research Centre of Canada after a double-blind, placebo-controlled study. [Arthritis Rheum. 2004 Oct. 15; 51 (5): 738-45.

SIDE EFFECTS AND INTERACTIONS
• May cause indigestion or nausea.

SAFETY CONCERNS
• Do not take if you have an allergy to shellfish.

DOSAGE

1,500 mg per day. It's often combined with chondroitin, also believed to nourish cartilage.

Green Tea

Common uses:
To lower the risk of cancer and other chronic diseases; to treat and prevent rheumatoid arthritis.

Green tea contains anti-oxidant compounds called polyphenols that reduce inflammation and protect against cancer. It's been used medicinally in Asia for thousands of years. Green tea may protect against heart disease by lowering cholesterol and blood pressure; increase longevity; prevent tooth decay (the tea contains fluoride); and help heal gum infections.

SCIENTIFIC EVIDENCE

Several studies suggest that the polyphenols in green tea reduce the inflammation of rheumatoid arthritis. One study suggests it not only reduces inflammation but also slows cartilage breakdown. [J Nutr. 2002 Mar; 132 (3): 341-6.] In a study on mice with induced arthritis at Case Western Reserve University in Cleveland, the mice give green tea polyphenols had a 33-55 percent lower incidence of arthritis compared with the placebo group. And in those who did have arthritis, the symptoms were less severe. [Proc Natl Acad Sci U S A 1999 Apr 13; 96 (8):

4524-9.] A number of studies suggest green tea may prevent cancer as well. In fact, green tea is now an established cancer preventive drink in Japan. [Cancer Lett. 2002 Dec 15; 188 (1-2): 9-13.] In those who drink over ten cups of green tea a day, green tea has also been found to lower risk of heart disease. [Ann N Y Acad Sci. 2001 Apr; 928: 274-80.]

SIDE EFFECTS AND INTERACTIONS

- The caffeine in green tea may cause nervousness or sleeplessness.

- Caffeine can increase the effects of drugs such as tricyclic antidepressants, theophylline and supplements such as ephedra.

SAFETY CONCERNS

- Those with arthritis need to weigh possible benefit against the possibility of sleep disturbance. Pill form does not contain as much caffeine as the tea.

- Pregnant and nursing mothers should not drink green tea because of the caffeine.

DOSAGE

Three to four cups of tea a day, which contain a total of 200 to 320 mg of polyphenols. In extract or supplement form, take 100 to 300 mg per day.

Guaifenesin

Common uses:

To treat fibromyalgia and rheumatoid arthritis.

Guaifenesin is an expectorant used commonly in cough syrups and cold medicines. It works by thinning the mucus in the lungs. Originally it came from a tree bark extract called guaiacum and was used to treat arthritis in the 1500s. The theory behind its use for arthritis is that guaifenesin helps the kidneys excrete phosphates, preventing a buildup in the bones, muscles and tendons, which some believe interferes with the body's production of ATP, a molecule involved in energy release. But there's no scientific evidence to back the theory.

SCIENTIFIC EVIDENCE

No evidence has been established to support the idea that guaifenesin can treat arthritis. In an unpublished double-blind study in 1996, 20 women took 600 mg of guaifenesin twice a day. At the end of the study, there was no difference between the guaifenesin group and the placebo group. [Robert Bennett, MD; Paul St. Armand, MD]

SIDE EFFECTS AND INTERACTIONS

- May cause nausea and vomiting.

- May worsen arthritis symptoms for several months.

- Salicylates may block guaifenesin's effect. People who take the supplement need to avoid anything with salicylates, including plants, medications such as aspirin, topical ointments, supplements and some cosmetics or toiletries, including some deodorants, toothpastes, mouthwashes and makeup.

• Low blood sugar may interfere with the supplement's effectiveness. People with hypoglycemia should follow a low-carbohydrate diet.

SAFETY CONCERNS

• Pregnant and nursing women should not take guaifenesin.

DOSAGE

300 to 600 mg a day. You should be under the supervision of a physician while you are taking guaifenesin.

Guggul (Gugulipid)

Common uses:

To lower cholesterol and triglyceride levels; to help control arthritis-related inflammation.

Guggul comes from a tree native to India, the mukul myrrh tree. Its resin, gum guggul, inhibits the formation of plaque within arteries and lowers levels of fat and cholesterol. It may also lower inflammation from arthritis and even help people lose weight.

SCIENTIFIC EVIDENCE

Most studies focus on guggul's ability to reduce cholesterol, and most, but not all, are promising. One study of those with high cholesterol showed no effect after eight weeks of therapy and in fact LDL levels (bad cholesterol) rose. [JAMA. 2003 Aug 13; 290 (6): 765-72.] In two clinical multi-center trials, patients who took guggul lowered their cholesterol and triglycerides significantly. [J Assoc Physicians India. 1989 May; 37 (5): 323-8.] Researchers at Baylor College of Medicine in Texas showed in animal studies that guggul aids the excretion of excess blood fats. [Science. 2002 May 31; 296 (5573): 1703-6. Epub 2002 May 02.] Although research is scant regarding guggul and arthritis, a study at Southern California University of Health Sciences showed that guggul significantly improved symptoms in those with osteoarthritis of the knee. [Altern Ther Health Med. 2003 May-Jun; 9 (3): 74-9.]

SIDE EFFECTS AND INTERACTIONS

- May cause nausea, gas, diarrhea, hiccups, restlessness, anxiety or headaches, though rarely.

SAFETY CONCERNS

- If you suffer from liver disease, inflammatory bowel disease or diarrhea, consult your doctor before taking.

- Do not take if you are pregnant.

- Buy only products marked as a gugulipid supplement and not as guggul or guggulu. The crude form could contain toxic compounds.

DOSAGE

25 mg guggulsterones three times daily.

Guided Imagery

Common uses:
To reduce pain and stress.

Guided imagery is the practice of creating mental images that induce relaxation and relieve stress, with the help of a practitioner or audiotape. The process also boosts the immune system and reduces pain. In theory, the practice works because the body perceives the induced image as the real experience. If you imagine yourself on a sunny beach relaxing, your body will in fact relax, your pulse slow, your blood pressure drop, and you will also release endorphins, the body's natural painkillers. A session with a practitioner may begin with his asking you about places that make you feel happy. Next, he will lead you through a series of relaxation or breathing exercises, then a visualization exercise asking you to pick images important to you. For example, you may want to picture yourself free of pain or full of energy. With practice, you can learn to do such exercises on your own throughout the day whenever you are feeling stressed.

SCIENTIFIC EVIDENCE

Hundreds of studies have proven that guided imagery works in lowering stress, decreasing stress and boosting the immune system. And it addresses these areas whether patients have arthritis, cancer or even asthma. For example, when women with osteoarthritis listened to guided imagery tapes twice a day in 10-15 minutes segments, they experienced significant reductions in pain and an increase in mobility over 12 weeks compared to the control group. [Pain Manag Nurs. 2004 Sep; 5(3): 97-104.] In a pilot study involving adults with asthma, almost half the patients using imagery were able to reduce or discontinue their medication compared to 19 percent of the control group. [Altern Ther Health Med. 2004 Jul-Aug; 10(4): 66-71.] In a small study of children with rheumatoid arthritis who were taught relaxation exercises twice a week for four weeks, their pain was substantially reduced, and they had increased functioning over 12 months. [Pediatrics. 1992 Jun: 89 (6 Pt l): 1075-9.] In a controlled clinical trial of cancer patients, those who received relaxation and imagery training reported reduced pain compared to the placebo group. [Pain. 1995 Nov; 63(2): 189-98.]

SIDE EFFECTS AND INTERACTIONS

- People with mental illness should talk with their therapist before using guided imagery.

SAFETY CONCERNS

- Let your practitioner know if you have nightmares or disturbing memories as the result of guided imagery.

FINDING A PRACTITIONER

Practitioners are not required to be licensed or certified. The best way to find someone is to ask your doctor for a referral. Wellness centers and hospitals also offer classes or attend an Arthritis Self-Help Course. Check the credentials of any practitioner you plan to work with. Or contact the Academy for Guided Imagery, (800) 726-2070, or www.interactiveimagery.com.

Heat/Cold Treatments

(See also hydrotherapy, p. 138)

Common Uses:

To decrease pain and increase flexibility.

Heat increases blood flow by dilating small blood vessels in the treated area, offering nourishment to the tissues, which speeds healing. Heat also relaxes muscles, lessening pain and muscle spasm. Heat can be applied through hot compresses, heat lamps, heating pads, whirlpool baths and hot tubs. Ultrasound reaches deeper joints and muscles than the other therapies.

Cold treatments help decrease blood flow and relieve short-term joint pain and swelling. Cold treatments can be in the form of ice packs, compresses or packs of frozen vegetables. Cold may be better for chronic pain (pain lasting longer than 14 days).

SCIENTIFIC EVIDENCE

Studies are inconsistent. Most studies of heat and cold therapies for arthritis show some relief of pain, stiffness and an increase in joint function. A Croatian study found that the pain threshold in patients using warm baths and ice massage was raised by both therapies. [Z Rheumatol. 1993 Sept-Oct; 52 (5): 289-91.] But in-vitro studies show that heat increases the breakdown of cartilage and tissues that contain collagen. [Semin Arthritis Rheum. 1994)ct; 24 (2): 82-90.] In a review of seven studies and 328 subjects with rheumatoid arthritis, reviewers found that heat and cold therapies had no significant effect on disease activity but did pro-vide short-term relief. [Cochrane Database Syst Rev. 2002 (2): CD002826.]

SIDE EFFECTS AND INTERACTIONS

None

SAFETY CONCERNS

• Don't use heat with topical rubs or creams like capsaicin since this cause skin burns.

DOSAGE

Apply treatments 4-6 times per day for 20-minute ses-sions.

Homeopathy

Common uses:

To stimulate the body to heal itself.

Homeopathy is one of most widely used complemen-tary therapies. It was developed in the 18th century when a German doctor, Samuel Hahnemann, discovered that quinine, a drug for malaria, produced malaria-like symptoms in healthy people. He became convinced that a very small amount of the very substances that caused an illness in a healthy person could create a healing response in a sick one. Treatment consists of giving remedies that will create the same symptoms as the disease. And the belief is that the weaker the remedy, the stronger the healing reaction. It's unclear why this may or may not work.

SCIENTIFIC EVIDENCE

Homeopathic treatment is tough to assess scientifically since it involves what researchers call "a package of individualized care," including consultation (a vital part of homeopathy) and medication. A review of six trials using homeopathic treatment to address asthma concluded that there was not enough evidence to assess homeopathy's role. [Respir Med. 2004 Aug; 98 (8): 687-96.] A review of homeopathic care in Germany suggests that homeopathy has more effect than placebo. But the researchers also recognize the studies' weaknesses and inconsistencies. [J Altern Complement Med. 1998 Winter; 4 (4): 371-88.] In a small trial of 23 people with rheumatoid arthritis, researcher found that homeopathic remedies relieved pain, stiffness and grip compared to placebo. [Br J Clin Pharmacol. 1980 May; 9 (5): 453-9.] But a six-month, double-blind British study of patients with rheumatoid arthritis found no evidence that homeopathy improved symptoms of rheumatoid arthritis.

SIDE EFFECTS AND INTERACTIONS

- Do not take homeopathic remedies if you are pregnant or an alcoholic since many of the remedies are in a base of alcohol and water.

SAFETY CONCERNS

- The risks are small because the remedies are so diluted (typically in alcohol and water). And they are regulated as over-the-counter drugs by the FDA.

- Do not use to treat a life-threatening illness.

- Do not stop prescribed medication to use homeopathy without consulting your doctor.

FINDING A PRACTITIONER

Only a few states have homeopathic licensing laws: Arizona, Nevada and Connecticut. Homeopathy is part of the training for naturopathic physicians. Look for someone who has been through a homeopathic training or certification program. Ask your doctor for a referral. Also, contact the National Center for Homeopathy, (877) 624-0613 or (703) 548–7790, or at www.homeopathic.org..

DOSAGE

Follow the instructions on whatever homeopathic remedy you are using. Do not keep taking once you have recovered or if you have not improved after a week.

Horsetail

Common uses:

Used as a diuretic and as a remedy for bladder and kidney problems.

Horsetail is a plant with long bamboo-like stems – the part used as medicine – and brown cones that give the plant its name. In the past, horsetail was used to control bleeding from lung lesions caused by tuberculosis. And in fact, animal studies show it does help staunch external bleeding. Currently, horsetail is used as a diuretic or to treat kidney and bladder problems. Several compounds – equisetonin and flavone glycosides – promote fluid loss. It also has anti-inflammatory qualities, making it useful for treating gastrointestinal conditions like Crohn's disease. It contains silica as well, which helps strengthen nails, hair and teeth – and may help address baldness. The body also uses silica to keep connective tissue and joint cartilage strong, making it useful in preventing osteoporosis and in treating bursitis and tendonitis.

SCIENTIFIC EVIDENCE

Studies do indicate that horsetail acts as a diuretic but there has only been limited research on humans. One study suggests that horsetail increases the rate of bone formation and encourages the deposit of calcium into bones. But the study is too small and flawed to indicate any benefit for those with osteoporosis. A Spanish study of seven plants including horsetail found that it was of some benefit in preventing and treating kidney stones in rats. [Int Urol Nephrol. 1994; 26 (5): 507-11.]

SIDE EFFECTS AND INTERACTIONS

- Do not take with diuretic medications.

- Horsetail contains a small amount of nicotine so don't take it if you are wearing nicotine replacement patches.

- Drink plenty of water while you are taking horsehair.

SAFETY CONCERNS

- Large doses can cause problems because of the nicotine Stop taking and call your doctor if you experience muscle weakness, a fast or irregular heartbeat, or other discomforts.

- Do not take to reduce swelling from poor kidney or heart function.

DOSAGE

Steep one tablespoon dried herb in one cup hot water. Add a little sugar to release silica from the leaves. Drink up to three times daily. If you use the extract, as one half teaspoon to a glass of water three times a day. Or take in capsule form, also three times a day.

Hydrotherapy

Common uses:

To reduce pain, stiffness and inflammation.

Hydrotherapy is the use of water – hot or cold – to treat disease and injury. The therapy includes anything from hot packs to baths, from whirlpools to wraps. It can include exercise programs in hydrotherapy pools, whirlpool baths and swimming pools. Hot hydrotherapy relieves tense muscles; cold helps decrease inflammation. The motion of a whirlpool has a relaxing, massage-like effect. Whirlpools are particularly soothing for those with arthritis.

Contrast hydrotherapy uses alternating hot and cold treatments to stimulate circulation. For instance, a 30-minute bath, alternating four minutes of heat and one minute of cold can increase blood flow by 90 percent.

The easiest form of hydrotherapy, of course, is a hot bath. For those with fibromyalgia, a hot bath can soothe sore muscles and also improve sleep. The water should be no hotter than 110 degrees Fahrenheit.

Cold helps relieve pain, particularly after overexertion or exercise. Fill a plastic bag with ice or use a bag of frozen vegetables, wrap in a towel, and apply to the painful spot for 20 minutes. Wait 20 minutes between applications.

Balneotherapy is a specialized kind of hydrotherapy involving water full of minerals such as sulphur, or mineral-rich mud.

SCIENTIFIC EVIDENCE

A number of studies show the effectiveness of hydrotherapy in relieving arthritis symptoms, although some researchers note that the studies are too flawed to draw definite conclusions. [Forsch Komplementarmed Klass Naturheilkd. 2004 Feb; 11 (1): 33-41. In a study of 50 patients with fibromyalgia, the group that had pool-based exercise had longer lasting and more thorough relief than those who had balneotherapy without exercise. [Rheumatol Int. 2004 Sep; 24 (5): 272-7. Epub 2003 Sep 24.] A review of six balneotherapy trials involving patients with rheumatoid arthritis concluded that despite positive results, the studies were flawed. [Cochrane Database Syst Rev. 2003 (4): CD000518] In a randomized, controlled trial comparing gym-based and hydrotherapy-based strengthening programs for those with osteoarthritis, researchers found function improved in both groups, although the gym-based group gained greater strength. [Ann Rheum Dis. 2003 Dec; 62 (12): 1162-7.]

SIDE EFFECTS AND INTERACTIONS

None

SAFETY CONCERNS

- Hot immersion baths, whirlpool spas, and saunas are not recommended for people with diabetes, high or low blood pressure, or for pregnant women.

- Do not heat a compress in a microwave. It can get too hot. Heat with hot water instead.

- Wrap ice in a towel before applying a cold pack.

- Do not combine hot and cold treatments with topical ointments like capsaicin, or you may burn yourself.

- Do not use cold treatments if you have Raynaud's phenomenon.

DOSAGE

Make hot baths no longer than 15 minutes at no warmer than 115 degrees Fahrenheit. Apply cold treatments for 20 minutes. Wait 20 minutes before retreating.

FINDING A PRACTITIONER

Most hospitals and medical centers offer some form of hydrotherapy. Ask your doctor to refer you to a program. Naturopaths are also trained in hydrotherapy.

Hypnosis

Common uses:

To relieve pain, anxiety; to treat irritable bowel syndrome; to alter behavioral habits such as smoking or overeating.

Hypnosis, also called hypnotherapy, is a kind of focused attention and deep relaxation. Modern hypnotism began in the late 18th century when an Austrian doctor named Franz Anton Mesmer, who treated patients with magnets, was thought to "mesmerize" his subjects. Hypnosis is used to change behavior and thinking, and its therapy can lower blood pressure, decrease heart rate and slow brain activity. Hypnosis will not make you go into a trance; it only allows you to focus more intently, augmenting the effect of mind-body techniques like relaxation exercises or visualization. Sessions begin with a relaxation exercise, followed by suggestions related to your therapeutic goals.

SCIENTIFIC EVIDENCE

In 1995, a National Institutes of Health panel recommended that hypnosis be part of medical treatment for chronic pain. There hasn't been much research regarding hypnotherapy and arthritis. However, a 1991 clinical trial found that fibromyalgia patients treated with hypnosis for 12 weeks had significantly more improvement in pain, fatigue, and sleep than a group treated with physical therapy. [J Rheumatol. 1991 Jan; 18 (1): 72-5.] And a number of studies suggest its effectiveness in treating pain generally, as well as irritable bowel syndrome. Scientists believe hypnosis may work by affecting the cortex, a part of the brain that affects how pain is experienced.

SIDE EFFECTS AND INTERACTIONS

None

SAFETY CONCERNS

- Hypnosis doesn't work on everyone. Do not continue treatment if you don't see results.

- Don't try hypnosis if you suffer from psychosis, a psychiatric condition, or an antisocial personality disorder.

- Do not substitute hypnosis for medical treatment of an illness.

FINDING A PRACTITIONER

Hypnotists are not licensed or regulated, so it's best to get a referral from your doctor or from a practitioner you trust. You can also contact the following:

- The National Guild of Hypnotists
  (603) 429-9438
  www.ngh.net

- American Council of Hypnotist Examiners
  (818) 242-1159
  www.hypnotistexaminers.org

K-m

Kava Kava

Common uses:

Treating anxiety and pain; as a muscle relaxant or sleep aid.

Kava kava is a member of the pepper family that grows in the Pacific Islands and Hawaii, where it has been used as a drink for special occasions and religious ceremonies. It has a relaxing effect without the stupor, say, of alcohol and drugs, and it is not addictive. Researchers aren't certain how kava works but believe it affects the limbic system, which controls emotion. Unfortunately, reports of liver damage have prompted the FDA to issue a warning about kava. Some practitioners believe short-term doses are not dangerous but others warn against taking it.

SCIENTIFIC EVIDENCE

A number of studies show that kava is effective for anxiety. [Jour Clin Psychopharmacol 2000; (1): 84]. No research exists on kava and arthritis per se. However, a number of studies point to its relaxing effects on muscles, which may relieve muscle spasms and pain. Others suggest it promotes sleep.

SIDE EFFECTS AND INTERACTIONS

- May cause upset stomach. Long-term use may cause dry, scaly, yellow skin.

- May increase drowsiness caused by drugs that affect

the central nervous system such as antidepressants, tranquilizers, sedatives, alcohol and herbs such as valerian.

• May increase the effects of MAO inhibitors and of herbs that act like MAO inhibitors such as evening primrose oil.

• May enhance effects of anesthesia. Do not take three weeks before surgery.

• Do not take with any medication that affects the liver, including acetaminophen (*Tylenol*).

SAFETY CONCERNS

• There have been reports of liver damage and death caused by doses once believed safe. It's best to avoid kava altogether. If you do take it, do so only under the supervision of a doctor.

• Do not take kava if you have a liver disease.

• Do not take if you have Parkinson's disease; it can aggravate symptoms.

• Do not take if you are pregnant or nursing.

• Fatigue, nausea, yellow skin, dark urine, yellowing of the eyes and light-colored stools are signs of liver toxicity. Stop kava immediately if you experience any of these signs.

DOSAGE

Do not take kava; it has been associated with liver toxicity and death.

Kinesiology Chiropractic (Applied Kinesiology)
(See also chiropractic, p. 75)

Common uses:

To diagnose and treat health problems by identifying weakened muscles.

Kinesiology chiropractic is a completely different field than conventional kinesiology. Kinesiology is the study of anatomy in relation to movement; its students usually work in physical therapy. Applied kinesiology is practiced by chiropractors, some osteopaths, and MDs with specific postgraduate training. Only licensed health-care professionals can get certification in kinesiology chiropractic.

The practice was developed in the 1960s. It is based on the idea that changes in muscle function occur as the result of internal triggers such as injury, pinched nerves, skeletal misalignment, nutritional deficiencies or even emotional issues. Through muscle testing, the practitioner finds the internal trouble spot and plans a health regimen based on that. The plan could include anything from chiropractic to diet changes. There has been no evidence establishing applied kinesiology as effective.

SCIENTIFIC EVIDENCE

Virtually all the scientific exploration of kinesiology chiropractic is either inconclusive or indicates that the therapy is ineffective. Most suggestions for use are based on tradition or scientific theory.

SIDE EFFECTS AND INTERACTIONS

None

SAFETY CONCERNS

• Kinesiology chiropractic should never replace conventional diagnosis or treatment.

• Ask to see the credentials of any practitioner you plan to use.

FINDING A PRACTITIONER

Ask your doctor for a referral to a health-care practitioner who has advanced certification in kinesiology chiropractic. You can also go to the International College of Applied Kinesiology website for referrals to practitioners, (913) 384-5336; www.icaksusa.com.

Lavender

Common uses:
Treating anxiety, sleeplessness, pain, digestive difficulties

Lavender is a flowering evergreen shrub native to the Mediterranean with a long history of medicinal use. The scent is thought to be relaxing, and Romans used it to freshen their baths.

SCIENTIFIC EVIDENCE

A number of studies suggest that lavender has a relaxing

effect. In a clinical trial in Japan, young women soaking their feet in hot water combined with lavender oil showed lowered autonomic responses consistent with relaxation. [Complement Ther Med. 2000 Mar; 8 (1): 2-7.] A clinical trial in England reported that patients in intensive care had improved moods and less anxiety after aromatherapy with lavender oil. [J Adv Nurs. 1995 Jan; 21 (1): 34-40.] But a clinical trial of patients undergoing radiotherapy found that aromatherapy was no help in reducing anxiety. [J Clin Oncol. 2003 June 15; 21 (12): 2372-6.

Several animal studies suggest that lavender – in particular, a component of lavender, perillyl alcohol – taken internally reduces some kinds of cancer growth. In studies at the University of Wisconsin at Madison, the growth of mammary tumors in rats fed perillyl alcohol slowed. [Clin Cancer Res 2000; 6(2): 390].

SIDE EFFECTS AND INTERACTIONS

- May cause a skin rash.

- May cause nausea, headaches and chills after inhaling.

- In large doses, perillyl alcohol can cause constipation, drowsiness and confusion.

- Taken internally, lavender may increase the drowsiness induced by drugs such as *Valium*, *Ativan*, barbiturates, narcotics, antidepressants, antihistamines and alcohol. It can do the same with some herbs such as valerian, chamomile or kava.

- May increase the risk of bleeding when taken with anticoagulants.

- May increase the cholesterol-lowering effect of some drugs and supplements.

SAFETY CONCERNS

- Do not take lavender internally if you are pregnant or nursing.
- Do not take internally without consulting your doctor.

DOSAGE

For aromatherapy, use five to seven drops of essential oil of lavender in bath water; or two to four drops in three cups of boiling water (for inhaling the steam). Use one to two teaspoons of dried lavender flowers to one cup of water for tea.

Leeches

Common uses:
To relieve the pain of osteoarthritis of the knee; to drain blood around skin grafts.

Leech therapy is used in Ayurvedic medicine, and it's a widespread treatment for knee pain in Germany. Analgesic and anesthesizing components in the leech saliva may produce the effect. In the past several decades, doctors have also found leeches useful in draining excess blood from serious wounds such as those created by skin grafts. Leeches secrete hirudin, a blood thinner that breaks up the blood helping it drain from the wound, which in turn allows normal blood vessels to form. Indian researchers have had some success using leeches on varicose veins.

SCIENTIFIC EVIDENCE

In 2001, German scientists found that four leeches placed on the painful osteoarthritic knees of ten patients for one hour resulted in 30 days of reduced pain. Those who had conventional therapy experienced no relief. The theory is that the leech saliva, which contains anesthetic and analgesic compounds, could have produced the result. [Annals of the Rheumatic Diseases. Dis, Nov. 4, 2003; 139 (9): 724-7300.]

In 2004, the FDA approved the marketing of leeches for medicinal purposes.

SIDE EFFECTS AND INTERACTIONS

- The "yuck" factor: Applying slimy creatures to skin may seem unpleasant to some people.

SAFETY CONCERNS

- Possible infection.

DOSAGE

The researchers and doctors who have used leeches for therapy used several leeches at a time for an hour or more. In the case of blood draining, the leeches fill with blood and drop off after several hours and must be replaced.

FINDING A PRACTITIONER

Right now, leeches are only being used in studies or in specific circumstances like skin grafting. It may be difficult to find a practitioner.

Lipase

Common uses:

To help the body absorb food more easily; to treat autoimmune disorders such as rheumatoid arthritis and lupus; also celiac disease, indigestion, foods allergies and cystic fibrosis.

Lipase is a digestive enzyme that breaks down fats, particularly triglycerides, so that they are more easily absorbed into the intestines. Lipase is produced primarily by the pancreas, but also in the mouth and stomach. Lipase supplements in tablets or capsules are usually from animal enzymes although there are also plant lipases available.

SCIENTIFIC EVIDENCE

Although no studies have been done connecting lipase supplements to relief of rheumatoid arthritis or lupus, some clinicians prescribe it. Pancreatic insufficiency, a condition in which the pancreas does not secrete enough chemicals and enzymes for normal digestion, frequently occurs in lupus, cystic fibrosis, ulcers, celiac disease and Crohn's disease. According to a study at the Oklahoma University College of Medicine, people with lupus, rheumatoid arthritis or Sjögren's syndrome often have antibodies to lipase, which in the lupus patients may contribute to high triglyceride levels. [Arthritis Rheum. 2002 Nov; 46 (11): 2957-63] More studies exist indicating lipase's role in digestion and celiac disease. In a double-blind study, subjects who stuffed down almost 1,200 calories of high-fat cookies experienced significant relief in bloating and fullness after taking lipase, a response that could be helpful to those with irritable bowel syndrome. [Dig Dis Sci. 1999 Jul; 44 (7): 1317-21.] In children with celiac disease, those treated with lipase had significantly higher weight gain (a good thing) compared to those treated with placebo. [Dig Dis Sci. 1995 Dec; 40 (12): 2555-60.]

SIDE EFFECTS AND INTERACTIONS

- Orlistat (*Xenical*), a medication used to treat obesity, blocks the action of lipase.

SAFETY CONCERNS

- None reported.

DOSAGE

One to two capsules of 6,000 LU (Lipase Activity Units) three times daily.

Low Energy Laser Therapy (Cold Laser Therapy)

Common uses:

To treat osteoarthritis; to increase speed, quality and strength of tissue repair; to relieve pain and inflammation.

Low energy laser therapy was introduced about ten years ago as a treatment for osteoarthritis. But it's still unclear how effective it is. The therapy is the application of red or near infrared light over injuries to improve healing and relieve acute and chronic pain. Red light increases the production of ATP, the body's molecules that story energy, which offers the cell more energy for healing.

SCIENTIFIC EVIDENCE

Research is increasingly showing laser therapy's effectiveness. But many of the early studies lacked proper controls. A Cochrane review of five trials found that, although there were some positive effects, it was unclear which factors of the treatment had the effect: wavelength, duration, dosage or site of application (nerves instead of joints). [The Cochrane Library, Issue 2, 2004.] But another review of 14 trials found that patients' chronic joint pain was cut in half compare to no change in the control group. [Australian Journal of Physiotherapy 2003. 49: 107-116.] Another study showed pain halved for 10 weeks. [Lasers in Surgery and Medicine 203 33: 330-338.]

SIDE EFFECTS AND INTERACTIONS

None

SAFETY CONCERNS

- You should wear goggles to prevent any harm to your eyes.

- If you are pregnant, you should not expose any area surrounding the fetus to laser therapy. Male genitals and malignancies should also not be exposed.

DOSAGE

Treatments can last from seconds to minutes. Studies indicate that it may be more effective to receive lower doses at multiple intervals than treatment with a single large dose.

FINDING A PRACTITIONER

Ask your doctor for a referral to a doctor trained in laser therapy.

Magnesium

Common uses:

To maintain muscle and nerve function; to keep heart rhythm regular; to strengthen teeth and bones; to alleviate premenstrual syndrome; to reduce fatigue and insomnia.

Low levels of magnesium are linked to osteoporosis; high blood pressure, heart attacks, strokes, diabetes and migraines. The mineral is found in artichokes, oatmeal, wheat germ, brown rice, almonds, cashews, hazelnuts, sunflower seeds, beans, Swiss chard and mineral water. Magnesium is considered a natural tranquilizer that relaxes skeletal muscles as well as the muscles of blood vessels and the gastrointestinal tract.

SCIENTIFIC EVIDENCE

Many effects of magnesium deficiency have been verified by studies. In a Canadian study, patients with rheumatoid arthritis were found to lack magnesium, a finding replicated in other studies. [Journal of Rheumatology (Canada), 1996, 23/6 (990-994)] And stress, an emotional and physical factor in arthritis, increases the need for magnesium. [J Am Coll Nutr (USA) Oct 1994, 13 (5) p429-46.]

SIDE EFFECTS AND INTERACTIONS

- Excess can cause diarrhea, confusion, muscle weakness, nausea, irregular heartbeat and low blood pressure.
- May make some antibiotics less effective.

SAFETY CONCERNS

- See Side Effects above.

DOSAGE

Do not take more than 350 mg daily in supplement form. Acidity aids absorption so take magnesium between meals or before bed.

Magnet Therapy

Common uses:

Relieving pain.

Magnet therapy has been used for centuries. In fact, some say Cleopatra even used magnets. Although no one knows how they work (or even if they work), in theory, the magnetic fields of the magnets penetrate the body, increasing circulation around painful areas or interfering with pain signals. Therapeutic magnets are many times stronger than household magnets. Magnet strength is measured in gauss. A refrigerator magnet is about 60 gauss. Therapeutic magnets range from 300 to 4,000 gauss. They come in strips that can be attached to the body, shoe insoles, mattress pads or car seats. The costs can range from $25 for a small magnet to $800 for a magnetic mattress pad. Low-level magnets are not effective.

SCIENTIFIC EVIDENCE

Early studies have been mixed but recent studies have been more positive, at least in treating arthritis. In a double-blind, placebo-control trial, patients with osteoarthritis of the knee had significantly less knee pain than the placebo group after six weeks. [Altrn Ther Health Med. 2004 Mar-Apr; 10 (2): 36-43.] Another double-blind clinical study showed that those with osteoarthritic knees had considerably less pain after treatment sessions than the placebo group. [Altern Ther Health Med. 2001 Sep-

Oct; 7 (5): 54-64, 66-9] And fibromyalgia patients who slept on magnetic pads for six months had significantly less pain than the placebo group, but remained similar to the placebo group in the number of tender points they reported and in their ability to function. [J Altern Complement Med. 2001 Feb; 7 (1): 53-64]

SIDE EFFECTS AND INTERACTIONS

- You may feel tingling in the part of the body closest to the magnet.

- If magnets do increase circulation, they may cause medications to be absorbed more quickly so watch for any changes in how you feel.

SAFETY CONCERNS

- Do not use if you are pregnant.

- Do not use if you have a pacemaker or implanted defibrillator, or if you are near anyone with those devices.

- Do not sleep on a magnetic mattress pad for more than eight hours.

- Turn off any electrical equipment such as electric blankets that may be sensitive to magnetic fields.

DOSAGE

Therapeutic magnets range from 300 to 4,000 gauss. Therapy may be anywhere from five minutes to several hours a day.

FINDING A PRACTITIONER

Practitioners need no certification. It's best to get a referral to a therapist from your doctor or from an allopathic pain management specialist.

Manganese

Common uses:

To help combat arthritis; keep bones strong; reduce fatigue and irritability; improve muscle reflexes and memory.

Manganese is a naturally occurring metal that helps fight fatigue and jangled nerves, improve reflexes and boost memory. It also helps your body process glucosamine, a natural body substance that helps build and repair cartilage. Manganese is important for many functions including skeletal development; sex hormone production; digestion and conversion of food to energy. Foods high in manganese are bran, whole grains, nuts, leafy vegetables and wheat germ. Manganese deficiency is very rare.

SCIENTIFIC EVIDENCE

At least two recent studies demonstrate the effectiveness of manganese in treating osteoarthritis if used in combination with glucosamine and chondroitin. In a randomized placebo-controlled study of glucosamine, chondroitin and manganese, researchers found that that the combination was effective in treating mild to moderate osteoarthritis of the knee. [Osteoarthritis Cartilage. 2000 Sep; 8 (5): 343-50.] A 16-week randomized, double-blind, placebo-control crossover trial that also combined the three concluded that the combination relieves symptoms of osteoarthritis in the knee or low back. [Mil Med. 1999 Feb; 164 (2): 85-91.]

SIDE EFFECTS AND INTERACTIONS

- Oral contraceptives and antacids may interfere with manganese absorption.

- Manganese may inhibit the absorption of iron, copper and zinc.

SAFETY CONCERNS

- At high levels manganese can cause damage to the brain, liver, kidney and a developing fetus. Symptoms of overexposure include mental and emotional disturbances and clumsiness.

DOSAGE

Upper limit (UL) level is 11 mg for adults, including pregnant and nursing women.

Massage

Common uses:

To relieve pain, stress and stiffness.

Massage therapy is an ancient practice, used even by Hippocrates, the father of medicine, as early as 430 B.C.

It is part of Indian Ayurvedic medicine, and practiced in Europe and Asia as well. Doctors often recommend it for those with arthritis: it relaxes muscles, lessens pain, and helps relieve stress and tension. According to a 2003 survey by the American Massage Therapy Association, massage is the second most sought-after form of pain relief, following medication. Of those surveyed, one in five had received a massage within the past year, a 13-point jump since 1997.

There are more than 100 kinds of massage. Some of the more common forms include:

- Deep tissue massage: This method involves placing pressure on deep muscles and tissue, working in strokes across the grain, using fingers, thumbs and elbows. It can help tight muscles loosen but you can also feel sore afterwards.

- Myofascial release: Therapists apply gentle pressure to stretch the fascia, the connective tissue that covers muscles. It is often used for fibromyalgia.

- Reflexology: The therapist applies pressure with the tips of his fingers or thumbs to the feet, hands, and ears to improve function throughout the body. The theory is that energy flows through ten channels or zones ending in the hands or feet. And each zone links parts of the body to specific areas on the hands and feet. This gentle massage is a good choice for those who might find other massage painful.

- Shiatsu: Shiatsu also focuses on the flow of energy in the body. Body energy, or qi (pronounced chee) flows along pathways, or meridians, and illness is the result of blocked energy. As in acupuncture and acupressure, the therapist applies pressure to certain points on the meridians to restore energy flow.

- Skinrolling massage: The therapist gathers a roll of skin and moves across the underlying fascia to break adhesions that might be binding tissue layers and nerves. Although it can be very painful at first, some claim it offers long-lasting relief.

- Spray and stretch: The therapist applies a coolant spray like flouri-methane to a painful area and then gently stretches the muscles there. This is a therapy favored by physical therapists and medical doctors.

- Swedish massage: This is what most people think of as traditional massage. The therapist strokes, kneads and shakes muscles all over the body to relieve tightness. It increases circulation to muscles and joints and is also very relaxing.

- Trigger point therapy: The therapist applies strong finger pressure on specific spots to release knots of tension or pain. This can be painful if the pressure is too strong.

SCIENTIFIC EVIDENCE

The results of formal studies are equivocal, despite lots of anecdotal evidence that massage is helpful, at least in the short term. A 2002 review of studies founds that massage is particular helpful for back and neck pain when compared to placebo but not any more effective than physical therapy or exercise. [Med Clin North Am.

2002 Jan; 86 (1): 91-103.] A British review was more lukewarm, noting that results were promising but the evidence was not clear that massage could control pain. [Clin J Pain. 2004 Jan-Feb; 20 (1): 8-12.]

SAFETY CONCERNS

- Some types of massage can worsen high blood pressure, osteoporosis or circulation problems. Ask your doctors before trying.

- Do not have a massage if you are have a flare or are coming down with an illness. Do not massage areas where skin is broken, sore or painful

- Tell the therapist if you are pregnant.

FINDING A PRACTITIONER

Ask your physician to refer you to a therapist. Or you can contact one of the following institutions for a referral:

- The National Certification Board for Therapeutic Massage and Bodywork
  (800) 296-0664
  www.ncbtmb.com

- The American Massage Therapy Association
  (847) 864-0123
  www.amtamassage.org

Meditation

Common uses:

To relieve pain, stress and anxiety

Meditation is defined as an intentional but relaxed state of awareness. It has been practiced for centuries by many cultures including those of India and Asia. In the U.S. the closest practice to meditation is prayer. Meditation involves sitting in a quiet place and focusing on a single object, thought or sensation such as breath, a sound, a phrase or an image. Another form involves cultivating "mindfulness" or an awareness of the present moment. The approach, often used in stress reduction programs, may begin with a focus on breathing and expand to awareness of feelings throughout the body. In any form of meditation, if your attention wanders, you refocus and begin again. Research has confirmed that meditation can slow heart rate, lower blood pressure and the levels of stress hormones. Harvard University professor Herbert Benson has dubbed the effect "the relaxation response."

Some people find it hard to sit still long enough to learn a meditation technique. In that case, try meditating as you walk.

SCIENTIFIC EVIDENCE

A number of studies show that meditation can have healthful and long lasting results, decreasing activity in the sympathetic nervous system, the system that controls reaction to stress. Meditation decreases heart and breathing rates, lowers blood pressure and stress hormones, and relaxes brain waves. When 28 patients with fibromyalgia practiced mindful meditation weekly for eight weeks, they had a significant reduction in pain, fatigue and sleeplessness. They also had a lift in spirits and were able to function better. [Altern Ther Health Med. 1998 Mar; 4 (2): 67-70.] Another pilot study concluded that meditation (along with education and Qi Gong, a Chinese movement therapy) significantly lessened pain and tender points. [Arthritis Care Res. 2000 Aug; 13 (4): 198-204.] A similar study, however, indicated that the combination of meditation and Qi Gong was no more effective than an education support group. [J Rheumatol. 2003 Oct; 30 (1): 2257-62.]

SAFETY CONCERNS

- Meditation can raise powerful emotions so choose an experienced instructor.

- If you feel uncomfortable with one type of meditation or class, choose another.

FINDING A PRACTITIONER

Meditation instructors are not licensed or certified. Some mental health professionals incorporate meditation into their practices. And meditation is offered at some hospitals, and spiritual and meditation centers. Ask your instructor about his training before you begin.

Melatonin

Common uses:

To treat insomnia and jet lag.

Melatonin is a hormone produced by the pineal gland, which lies within the brain. Melatonin regulates sleep; the gland releases more melatonin when it's dark and less during daytime hours. As we age, the pineal gland secretes less melatonin.

Melatonin supplements are synthetic versions of the hormone. It is not addictive and is used to relieve insomnia and jet lag. Although people with fibromyalgia take melatonin to sleep better, people with auto-immune diseases like lupus should not use it. And its effects aren't clear so it should be taken under your doctor's supervision.

SCIENTIFIC EVIDENCE

Studies show that melatonin is effective for jet lag and for helping night workers adjust to new sleeping patterns. Other studies indicate it can be an effective sleep aid, especially in the elderly and in those with a low level of melatonin.

There are a number of studies that suggest melatonin levels plays a role in rheumatoid arthritis. In particular, they may have overly high nighttime levels of melatonin. In a review of animal studies, researchers concluded that low melatonin doses in rats with induced RA produced less alteration of 24-hour rhythms including those of the immune system, and less inflammation than in rats given high doses of melatonin. [Curr Drug Targets Immune Endocr Metabol Disord. 2004 Mar; 4 (1): 1-10.] [Neurosignals. 2003 Nov-Dec.; 12 (6): 267-82.]

Fibromyalgia patients who took melatonin for four weeks in a pilot study had less pain and improved sleep. [Clin Rheumatol. 2000; 19 (1): 9-13.] But another study indicated that fibromyalgia patients had significantly higher melatonin levels at night compared to those without fibromyalgia, leaving no reason for giving those with fibromyalgia melatonin supplements. [J Rheumatol. 1999 Dec; 26 (12): 2675-80.]

Side Effects and Interactions

- May cause drowsiness 30 minutes after taking.

- May cause headache, stomach upset, lethargy and disorientation.

- May induce post-nap grogginess, vivid or unpleasant dreams, and a worsening of insomnia.

- High doses may disturb your body clock and alter the production of other hormones. It may also affect a woman's menstrual cycle and fertility.

- Taken with sedatives, antihistamines, muscle relaxants, alcohol or narcotic pain relievers, melatonin may cause excessive drowsiness. The same is true if taken with herbs such as valerian, chamomile and kava.

- May increase blood pressure and heart rate in those taking antihypertensive medications.

SAFETY CONCERNS

- There is no evidence of its long-term safety. And because it is a hormone, it can have a number of effects. Talk to your doctor before taking, especially if you are taking other medications.

- Do not take it if you are also taking corticosteroids or birth control pills.

- If you have kidney disease, epilepsy, diabetes, depression, an auto-immune disease, serious allergies, heart disease, leukemia or multiple sclerosis, you should not take melatonin.

- Do not drive or do dangerous tasks while taking melatonin.

- Pregnant and nursing women should not take melatonin. Nor should children and teenagers.

- Buy synthetic melatonin only; melatonin from animal glands carry the risk of contamination.

DOSAGE

1mg before bedtime. However, start with a smaller dose; doses as low as 0.1mg are effective for some people.

Misai Kuching

Common uses:

To treat gout, arthritis, diabetes, kidney stones and hypertension; also used as a diuretic.

Misai kuching is an herb that grows in Malaysia that has been used as a remedy for centuries for everything from gout to kidney stones. It began to interest researchers at the start of the 20th century when it became popular in Europe as an herbal tea. It's thought to have an anti-inflammatory effect and to also flush out acids that inflame joints. Uric acid build-up is a major cause of gout, a painful form of arthritis where uric acid crystals collect and settle in joints such as the big toe.

SCIENTIFIC EVIDENCE

- Few scientific studies have been done on misai kuching. The most definitive Malaysian study suggests that the herb may be useful in inhibiting the formation and growth of kidney stones, in part by reducing the production of uric acid. [Sahabudin Raja Mohamed, Hospital Kuala Lumpur]

SAFETY CONCERNS

- None reported.

DOSAGE

Since so little research has been done on this herb, the dosage amount is unclear. People drink it as a tea.

MSM (methylsulfonylmethane)

Common uses:
To treat arthritis, back pain and muscle pain.

MSM is an organic sulfur compound found in the blood and most foods, and formed in the breakdown of DMSO. [See DMSO, p. tk]. Sulfur works with B vitamins to help nerve cells communicate. It's also an important nutrient for joints, and research suggests that people with arthritis may have low levels of sulfur in the joints. Other studies suggest that mineral baths high in sulfur help relieve arthritis symptoms. MSM itself is thought to have pain-relieving and anti-inflammatory properties, and it may help keep cartilage healthy. These qualities make it an attractive treatment for arthritis. However, there is little scientific evidence to support these claims.

SCIENTIFIC EVIDENCE

There is little evidence about MSM supplements; studies focus more often on the effects of sulphur in baths or nutrition. In a study of those with osteoarthritis, researchers found that three weeks of sulfur baths reduced oxidative stress and improved cholesterol readings compared to the control group. [Forsch Komplementarmed Klass Naturheilkd. 2002 Aug; 9 (4): 216-20.] A review of the role of sulphur in nutrition found sulfur a promising, safe treatment for a number of ailments including arthritis but also noted that human clinical trials are needed. [Altern

Med Rev. 2002 Feb; 7 (1): 22-44.] A double-blind study of the effect of MSM on those with degenerative arthritis found an 82 percent improvement in pain at the end of six weeks compared to an 18 percent improvement in the control group. [Ronald M. Lawrence, UCLA School of Medicine, 2001].

SIDE EFFECTS AND INTERACTIONS

- May cause upset stomach, diarrhea and headache.
- May cause rash.
- Should not be used with anticoagulants such as warfarin (*Coumadin*), aspirin, or blood-thinning supplements such as ginger or ginkgo biloba.
- Some experts advise those who have allergies to sulfa drugs and sulfites not to MSM. Others say it is safe.

SAFETY CONCERNS:

- The long-term effects are not known.

DOSAGE

500 mg two times a day taken with meals to avoid an upset stomach.

Myofascial Release

Common uses:
To relieve muscle tension, pain and emotional stress.

Myofascial release is form of massage and stretching in which therapists use gentle pressure to loosen the fascia, the connective tissue covering muscles. It is helpful for those with arthritis. The therapy is relatively new, begun by an osteopathic physician in the 1970s, although its roots go back to the soft-tissue manipulations of osteopathy. It's also considered an offshoot of Rolfing, a form of deep tissue bodywork begun in the 1930s. [See Rolfing, p. 203] For the past twenty years, practitioners such as physical therapists and chiropractors have adopted the method, using it as part of preventive care but also in pain management.

SCIENTIFIC EVIDENCE

Not a lot of research has been done on myofascial release, particularly on its relief of arthritis pain. However there are positive pain studies. A clinical trial found that in those with myofascial pain in the shoulder and upper back, this type of massage (along with several others) was effective in relieving trigger point pain and range of motion. [Arch Phys Med Rehabil. 2002 Oct.; 83 (10):1406-14.] A large clinical trial of those with low back pain found that those treated with osteopathic spinal manipulation, including myofascial release, required less pain medication that those receiving standard medical therapy. [N Engl J Med. 1999 Nov 4; 341 (19): 1426-31.] Many experts believe that myofascial release is not specific enough to relieve trigger point pain. Others feel it can be an effective treatment for arthritis.

SIDE EFFECTS AND INTERACTIONS

- Some people feel sore following treatment but it should resolves within a day or two.

- You may become nauseous or lightheaded during the treatment. Drink plenty of water following the treatment.

SAFETY CONCERNS

- If you have had recent surgery, an injury or are pregnant, let the therapist know before the session begins.

- If you take anticoagulants or bruise easily, also let the therapist know.

FINDING A PRACTITIONER

See Massage, p. 159.

Myotherapy (see neuromuscular massage, p. 176)

Naturopathic Medicine

Common uses:

To encourage healthy living habits, allowing the body to heal itself; to prevent disease.

Naturopathic medicine stems from the natural cures practiced in Europeans spas in the 19th century. Bernard Lust, who founded the American School of Naturopathy, introduced naturopathic medicine into the United States in 1896. Naturopathy became very popular until the rise of pharmaceutical and high-tech treatments after World War II. It is currently making a comeback; approximately 1,500 naturopathic physicians practice nationwide.

The principle behind naturopathy is one of prevention: the practice encourages exercise and good nutrition, relying on the body's ability to heal itself. The focus is on the individual, not the disease. A naturopath looks for causes of disease in a person's lifestyle and then recommends changes to eliminate those causes.

Naturopathic physicians receive four years of training that includes homeopathy, clinical nutrition, manipulation, herbal medicine and hydrotherapy. They are not licensed to perform surgery or to prescribe drugs.

SCIENTIFIC EVIDENCE

As this book attests, a number of studies on treatments that compose naturopathy suggest they can be effective treatments for arthritic pain.

SAFETY CONCERNS

- Naturopathic medicine is not meant to treat serious diseases, nor can naturopaths prescribe medication. If you have rheumatoid arthritis, lupus or other severe rheumatic diseases, your naturopath should refer you to a rheumatologist.

- Do not stop taking your medication without consulting your physician first.

- Make certain you are seeing a licensed naturopath (ND).

FINDING A PRACTITIONER

Naturopathic physicians (NDs) train for four years in homeopathy, nutrition, manipulation, herbal medicine, and hydrotherapy. The following organization can help you find a licensed practitioner:

- The American Association of Naturopathic Physicians
  (866) 538-2267
  www.naturopathic.org

Neuromuscular Massage

Common uses:
To release trigger point knots of tension and pain.

The therapy involves placing pressure for ten to 30 seconds on trigger point sites (specific knots or muscle spasms of tension and pain). Trigger points usually occur within a tight band of skeletal muscle in the fascia, the sheath that surrounds the muscles, and can cause pain in other parts of the body when they are compressed. As the muscle relaxes, lactic acid is released and circulation to the muscle increases. The therapy is painful at first, so it's important to tell the therapist if your treatment becomes too painful. But the pressure usually alleviates the muscle spasm. Resulting soreness should only last a day or two. Myotherapy (deep muscle massage and stretching) and trigger point therapy are forms of this type of massage.

Myotherapy grew out of myofascial trigger point therapy begun in the 1940s. It was more widely developed in the 1970s by health and exercise expert Bonnie Prudden. Prudden eventually developed the most widely know certification program for myotherapists.

Trigger Point Release Therapy is a system of neuromuscular massage therapy developed by the Colorado Institute of Massage Therapy. Therapists learn a number of techniques to release trigger points.

SCIENTIFIC EVIDENCE

The American Academy of Pain Management recognizes this therapy as an effective treatment for back pain caused by soft tissue injury such as muscle strain. And a number of studies have found massage in general to be an effective therapy for muscle-related pain. A randomized trial comparing acupuncture, therapeutic massage and self-care education found massage (which included trigger-point therapy and neuromuscular therapy) the most helpful at the end of ten weeks, with improvements that persisted for one year. [Archives of Internal Medicine, April 23, 200l, Vol. 161, N0. 8.]

SAFETY CONCERNS

- Do not use this therapy if you have a bleeding disorder that causes you to bruise easily.

- Do not apply pressure to a recent fracture, surgical incision or tumor.

- Avoid if you have any condition aggravated by deep pressure, such as a fibromyalgia flare.

FINDING A PRACTITIONER

Ask your doctor to refer you to a therapist who is certified in neuromuscular therapy. Myotherapists typically receive 1,300 hours of training; trigger point therapists 1,150 hours. For more information or help with referrals, contact:

- Bonnie Prudden Myotherapy, Inc.,
  (800) 221-4634
  www.bonnieprudden.com

- Colorado Institute of Massage Therapy
  (888) 634-7347
  www.coimt.com

Noni Juice

Common uses:

Preventing cancer; relieving pain, inflammation and digestive difficulties.

The noni plant is native to Indonesia where it has been used for thousands of years to treat a wide range of illnesses and symptoms. Although little research has been done on the plant, a number of in vitro and animal studies in recent years suggest it may prevent cancer. It also contains chemicals called anthraquinones that help relieve constipation.

SCIENTIFIC EVIDENCE

Over the past decade, researchers have focused on noni juice's potential as a cancer preventive. Researchers at the University of Hawaii in a series of studies (in vitro and with mice) showed that noni juice enhances the immune system, which in turn enables an attack on tumor cells. [Phytother Res. 2003 Dec; 17 (10): 1158-64.] It also appears noni juice has an analgesic effect. [Planta Medica 56 (1990). 430-434.] A more recent animal study also found noni to have pain-relieving, anti-inflammatory and anticancer properties. [Acta Pharmacol Sin. 2002 Dec; 23 (12): 1127]

SIDE EFFECTS AND INTERACTIONS

- Not much is known about its side effects. It may cause nausea and upset stomach.

- Noni may increase potassium in the body. People with kidney disease or who are taking potassium-sparing diuretics should not drink noni juice.

- Do not drink noni juice with coffee, tobacco or alcohol.

- The taste and smell of noni juice can be unpleasant. That's not true of the capsules, but drying noni fruit may change its effectiveness.

SAFETY CONCERNS

- Little is known about noni's safety. People with diabetes should avoid noni juice since its effect on blood sugar levels is unknown also.

- Pregnant and nursing women should avoid noni juice, again because its dangers are unknown.

DOSAGE

Four ounces on an empty stomach one half hour before breakfast.

Olive Leaf

Common uses:

To boost energy and the immune system; to improve heart health.

Olive leaf has been used for thousands of years to treat a range of ailments. The leaf is from the olive tree, a small evergreen common in the Mediterranean. The active ingredient in the plant is called oleuropein, which battles the replication of pathogens like viruses, bacteria and parasites. It may also lower blood pressure and cholesterol and ease blood flow. People with auto-immune forms of arthritis, such as RA, may be curious about olive leaf because of its purported immune-boosting properties.

SCIENTIFIC EVIDENCE

Several studies have found that olive leaf lowers blood pressure in animals. For instance in a study on hypertensive rats, olive extract returned their blood pressures to normal. [Arzneimittelforschung 2002; 52 (11): 797-802.] And Italian researchers have also found that the oleuropein in olive leaf kills a range of bacteria, fungi and viruses. [J Pharm Pharmacol 1999 Aug; 51 (8): 971-4] Yet another study found that oleuropein protects LDL, the good cholesterol, from oxidation, a process involved in heart disease. [Life Sci 1994; 55(24): 1965-71] European studies also suggest that olive leaf helps relax blood vessels, improving circulation, regulating heartbeat, and lowering both blood sugar and blood pressure. However, the bulk of studies have been animal or in vitro studies, and more studies are needed to test its effect on humans. Its effectiveness for boosting the immune system is unproven.

SIDE EFFECTS AND INTERACTIONS

None

SAFETY CONCERNS

- None reported.

- Do not take if you are pregnant or nursing.

DOSAGE

An effective amount hasn't been established. To make tea, steep one teaspoon of drive leaves in one cup hot water for 10-15 minutes.

Osteopathic Medicine

Common uses:

To treat all illness, with an emphasis on the musculoskeletal system.

Osteopathic medicine straddles complementary and conventional medicine. Its doctors (DOs) are educated in almost the same way as conventional MDs. They are licensed to perform surgery and to prescribe medications, and they can specialize in various fields. The differences lie in emphasis. Osteopaths view the musculoskeletal system as the seat of health so your treatment may involve manipulative therapy. Illness, osteopaths believe, upsets the balance in that system. And they also believe that blood flow helps most conditions, and that manipulation can improve blood flow. Osteopaths are particularly helpful to those with arthritis since their skills combine expertise with the musculoskeletal system and conventional medicine.

SCIENTIFIC EVIDENCE

Osteopathy is considered especially effective at treating back pain. [Journal of Manipulative & Physiological Therapeutics. 22 (2): 87-90, 1999 Feb.] But there have been few quality trials. A large clinical trial of low back pain and osteopathy (among other treatments) is currently under way in the UK. A study of 500 patients in an osteopathy practice found that those with acute symptoms did better than those with chronic symptoms. [British Journal of General Practice, 1993 Jan; 43 (366): 15-8.] Another pilot study compared those with low back pain who had osteopathic treatment plus management advice, and those who simply had management advice. Fifty percent of those who had osteopathic treatment had recovered after two weeks compared with 22 percent in the control group. That difference had lessened at the end of 12 weeks. [Spine Vol 15 No 5 May 1990]

SAFETY CONCERNS

- If your osteopath plans to use manipulation, tell him if you are having a flare or increased symptoms.

- You may be sore for a day or two after manipulation.

FINDING A PRACTITIONER

You can find an osteopath through most hospitals and health clinics. You can also contact the following for information and referrals:

- American Osteopathic Association
  (800) 621-1773
  www.osteopathic.org

Pau D'arco

Common uses:
To treat vaginal yeast infections; eliminate warts; to boost immunity.

Pau d'arco comes from the inner bark of an evergreen tree native to South and Central America. Although it was touted as possible treatment for cancer in the 1970s, its side effects – blood clots, anemia, nausea – were too severe for further human studies. Since then the most convincing evidence has centered on its antibacterial and antifungal powers. Some herbalists also feel it strengthens immunity, making it of interest to some people with auto-immune forms of arthritis.

SCIENTIFIC EVIDENCE

While there are no studies confirming many of the claims made for pau d'arco, researchers have found infection-fighting compounds in pau d'arco called napthoquinones, which kill certain bacteria, viruses and fungi. [Int J Antimicrob Agents. 2003 Mar; 21 (3): 279-84.] The antifungal property makes it effective for vaginal infections and other fungi-related conditions like athlete's foot and jock itch.

SIDE EFFECTS AND INTERACTIONS

• Pau d'arco can intensify anticoagulant medications.

• If it upsets your stomach, take it with foods. Stop taking it if it continues to cause upset.

SAFETY CONCERNS

• High doses can cause nausea, vomiting, excessive bleeding and other complications.

• Do not take for more than a week.

• Do not take if you are pregnant or breastfeeding.

DOSAGE

• For tea, use one teaspoon of loose, dried bark per one cup of water and boil for five to 15 minutes. Drink up to 8 times per day.

• Extract: Follow directions on the label.

• Tincture: Take 20 to 30 drops, two to three times a day.

• Capsules: l,000 mg three times a day.

Prayer

Common uses:

To help us cope with suffering and depression; to give comfort in illness and perhaps even aid healing.

Religion is a very important and private issue to many Americans. According to Gallup polls, 95 percent of us believe in God or a universal spirit. Two thirds of us pray at least once a day, and a third of us pray about our health. Government funding of prayer research began in the 1990s, and since 2000 at least ten studies have been carried out by places like the Mind/Body Medical Institute in Boston, Duke University and the University of Washington.

SCIENTIFIC EVIDENCE

The very abstraction of religion and faith makes it difficult to quantify its results in scientific studies. In many, researchers question whether the effect is due to religion and prayer per se or to increased social contact and positive attitudes that often accompany religious practice. Still, research suggests positive results. Several studies indicate that the positive use of religion can help deal with the stress of rheumatoid arthritis. [Arthritis Rheum. 2004 Feb 15; 51 (1): 49-55.] And a number indicate that people who attend religious services take better care of their health. [Am J Public Health. 1997 Jun; 87 (6): 957-61.] [Int J Psychiatry Med. 2002; 32 (1): 69-89.] A more recent study found frequent churchgoers had lower rates of chronic diseases like cancer than non-worshipers. [Int J Psychiatry Med. 2002; 32 (1): 69-89.] Another study found that in ill elderly patients, those who felt God had forsaken them or was punishing them had a 19 to 28 percent higher mortality rate than those without such a struggle. [Archives of Internal Medicine, 161, 1881-1885.] The association between religious involvement and depression is less clear. In a study of those with congestive heart failure, religious activity was associated with greater social support but only weakly related to less depression. [Journal of Religion and Health, 41 (3): 263-278.]

SAFETY CONCERNS

- Don't expect your religion to heal you, or feel that faith has failed you if your prayers for recovery aren't answered. The rewards of prayer stem from the process itself.

- Do not believe any spiritual leader who promises faith will heal you. And don't sign your savings over for that purpose.

DOSAGE

Of course, no one know what the effective "dosage" is when it comes to religion, which is one more factor that makes it tough to study and quantify.

Prolotherapy

Common uses:

To manage joint pain; to strengthen joints and ligaments.

The method has its origins in ancient times, when Hippocrates (the father of modern medicine) thrust a hot lance into the joint of injured javelin throwers' shoulders. The resulting scar tissue made the joint stronger. The modern version of the therapy began in an injection technique called sclerotherapy first used in the 1920s to treat hernias and hemorrhoids, a use expanded to back ailments in the '40s. The term *prolotherapy* began in the '50s to describe injections for pain management and for strengthening joints and ligaments.

The therapy works this way: After an injection of dextrose or saline into ligaments or tendons, the area becomes inflamed. The inflammation starts the body's healing response and promotes growth factors, which lay down new tissue and trigger the growth of new blood vessels and the flow of nutrients.

SCIENTIFIC EVIDENCE

Unfortunately studies to date have been inconclusive. In a 2004 review of seven studies, three had inadequate controls, two were too small to be conclusive, and two others had no control groups. Only case reports supported pursuing more controlled studies on the use of prolotherapy and chronic neck pain. [Am J Phys Med Rehabil.

2004 May; 83(5): 379-89.] Other reports are more positive. A small study of prolotherapy for osteoarthritic thumb and finger joints found it effective in the treatment of pain during movement. [J Altern Complement Med. 2000 Aug; 6 (4): 311-20.] And a double-blind study concluded that prolotherapy resulted in significant improvement in pain, swelling and movement for those with knee osteoarthritis. [Altern Ther Health Med. 2000 Mar; 6 (2): 68-74, 77-80.]

SIDE EFFECTS AND INTERACTIONS

- Avoid caffeine, alcohol and anti-inflammatory drugs during treatments. They may reduce the effectiveness of the treatments.

SAFETY CONCERNS

- Injections should only be given by a physician, osteopath or a naturopath (in states where licensed to do so) who has training in the technique.

FINDING A PRACTITIONER

There is no legal credentialing required since the method is included in any state medical license. Most doctors are trained by other doctors. You can also call the following training organizations for information or a referral.

- The American Association of Orthopaedic Medicine
  (800) 992-2063
  aaom@aaomed.org

- American College of Ostepathic Sclerotherapeutic Pain Management, Inc.
(302) 376-8080
http://acopms.com

Pulsed Electromagnetic Therapy

Common uses:

To stimulate healing of bone fractures and wounds; pain reduction.

A Swiss physician began magnetic therapy in the 16th century, using magnets to treat epilepsy, diarrhea and hemorrhage. Modern research suggests that the therapy can be effective in stimulating repair of bone fractures and soft tissue injury. The theory is that injury changes the electric impulses between cells and that a pulsating electromagnetic field helps return those impulses to normal. The therapy may address pain by blocking the pain signals via electric signal changes.

SCIENTIFIC EVIDENCE

Several studies suggest the therapy is effective at blocking pain signals. [Elsevier Biomedical Press, Pain Therapy 1983.] The USDA has approved the therapy for treating bone fractures. And the treatment's effectiveness is borne out by at least two double-blind studies. [J Bone and Joint Surg (BR) 72: 347-355, 1990.] [Spine 15: 708-712, 1990.] A contradictory study, however, shows delayed healing of fractures in rabbits when the therapy was used. [Clin Orthop 145: 245-51, 1979.] Other studies suggest it may be effective in healing chronic wounds. [J Orthop Res 8 (2): 276-282, 1990.] But a number of studies have drawn the opposite conclusion. [Lancet 8384 (1): 994-996, 1984.] Researchers also have concerns about the poor design of many studies and recommend further study.

SIDE EFFECTS AND INTERACTIONS

None

SAFETY CONCERNS

None

FINDING A PRACTITIONER

Get a referral from your doctor of someone trained in the therapy.

Q-s

Qi Gong

Common uses:
To promote health and self-healing.

Qi gong is an ancient system of meditation, breathing exercises and movement used to aid the flow of energy, or qi (pronounced chee) through the body. The exercises are fairly easy to do and can be done comfortably by those with arthritis – or even by someone in bed or a wheelchair. Classes begin with meditation and breathing exercises to help you quiet your mind and body so that you can focus on the flow of energy in your body. Ideally, qi gong should be practiced daily. It's thought that regular practice reduces stress and improves well-being. Although there are few verifying studies, practitioners believe it strengthens the immune system, decreases heart rate, lowers blood pressure and relieves pain.

SCIENTIFIC EVIDENCE

There are not a lot of English language studies about qi gong. Participants with fibromyalgia in a study at the University of Maryland combining qi gong with mindfulness meditation found their pain lessened, and their depression, coping skills and functioning improved, changes that lasted at least six months following the study. [Altern Ther Health Med. 1998 Mar; 4 (2): 67-70.]

A number of studies have found tai chi, a similar form of exercise, to be safe and effective. In a 2004 review of four trials involving 206 participants, researchers found that tai chi had no ill effects on those with rheumatoid arthritis and significantly improved range of motion, particular in the ankles. [Cochrane Database Syst Rev. 2004;(3):CD004849.] Yet another review of nine randomized controlled trials, 23 nonrandomized controlled studies, and 15 observational studies found tai chi benefits those with a range of chronic conditions including arthritis. Benefits included improvements in balance and strength, and flexibility. [Arch Intern Med. 2004 Mar 8;164(5):493-501. Review.] A randomized controlled clinical trial found that the symptoms in older women with osteoarthritis improved after 12 weeks of tai chi, as did their balance and function.[J Rheumatol. 2003 Sep;30(9):2039-44.]In a study of those with rheumatoid arthritis, tai chi was also found effective and safe. It may also help stimulate bone growth and strengthen connective tissue. [Am J Phys Med Rehabil. 1991 Jun; 70(3): 136-41.] It's likely these results would be similar for qi gong.

SIDE EFFECTS AND INTERACTIONS
None

SAFETY CONCERNS
- Don't overexert when doing these exercises. Most teachers agree that the focus on energy is more important than the physical exercise.

- If you are pregnant, do only mild exercise and only under the instruction of experienced teachers.

- Avoid if you have a tendency to become dizzy.

FINDING A PRACTITIONER

No certification is required so look for someone affiliated with a reputable health center. Also, the *Qi Journal* web site offers a list of teachers. www.qi-journal.com.

Quercetin

Common uses:
To reduce cancer risk, prevent heart attacks and cataracts; to ease asthma; to reduce inflammation from Crohn's disease; to prevent gout; to lessen heartburn.

Found in apples, onions, and black tea, quercetin is a flavonoid (plant pigment) and anti-oxidant that combats the free radical molecules that play a part in many diseases. Anti-oxidants are often cited as possibly preventing the joint and tissue damage that may be associated with arthritis. Quercetin also inhibits the buildup of a kind of blood sugar that leads to cataracts. It may also help prevent heart attacks.

SCIENTIFIC EVIDENCE

A number of studies suggest that quercetin may be effective in preventing heart disease. A 2002 study of 5,000 black tea drinkers showed that daily consumption reduced the risk of heart attack. [Am J Clin Nutr. 2002 May;75(5):880-6.] Researchers at Cornell have found that quercetin protects brain cells against oxidative stress, the tissue-damaging process associated with Alzheimer's disease. [C.Y. Lee,

Journal of Agricultural and Food Chemistry, 2004] A randomized, double-blind study indicated that daily doses of quercitin for 12 weeks increased healthy blood flow in the legs. [Arzneimettelforschung 50: 109-117.] A number of studies have shown its effectiveness in combating cancer as well. For instance, a Mayo Clinic research study showed that quercetin blocked hormone activity, which in turns helped prevent or stop prostate cancer cells. [Carcinogenesis, March 2001].

SIDE EFFECTS AND INTERACTIONS

- If you take hormone replacement therapy, quercetin may increase estradiol and reduce the effectiveness of other forms of estrogen.

- Don't take quercetin if you take felodipine, a calcium channel blocker.

SAFETY CONCERNS

None

DOSAGE

To prevent cancer, heart attack and cataracts, take 125-250 mg a day; for asthma, take 250-500 mg 3 times a day; for Crohn's disease, take 400 mg 3 times a day; for gout, 500 mg twice a day; for heartburn, 500 mg 3 times a day.

Reflexology

Common uses:
To relieve pain and stiffness.

Modern reflexology began in the early 1900s when American physician William H. Fitzgerald used gentle pressure on the hands and feet to stimulate health benefits in what he thought were corresponding zones in the body. The massages still center on points on the feet, hands, and ears – appealing choices when a full-body massage might be painful. The theory behind the therapy is that energy channels run vertically through the body. Because hands and feet have lots of nerve endings, stimulating them may affect other parts of the body. At the least, the therapy is relaxing.

SCIENTIFIC EVIDENCE

Although there are few studies about reflexology, some do indicate its benefits. In a study of 35 women with premenstrual syndrome (PMS), those treated with reflexology had more relief of their symptoms than the placebo group. [Obstet Gynecol. 1993 Dec; 82 (6): 906-11.] In another study of 220 Danish patients with tension or migraine headaches, 81 percent found that reflexology decreased or relieved their pain. [Altern Ther Health Med. 1999 May; 5 (3): 57-65.] And a number of Chinese studies show relief in those with arthritis. For instance, when 42 people with arthritis in their shoulders received foot reflexology treatments every day for 15 days, eight had no more pain, 14 improved, and 20 found it effective. [*Beijing International Reflexology Conference (Report)*, 1996, p. 55] Patients with lung and breast cancer had less anxiety after reflexology treatments, and the breast cancer patients had less pain. [Oncol Nurs Forum. 2000 Jan-Feb; 27 (1): 67-72.]

SAFETY CONCERNS

- Reflexologists are not qualified to diagnose or treat diseases.

- If you have a foot injury, blood clots, thrombosis, phlebitis or other vascular difficulties, talk to your doctor before trying reflexology.

- If you are pregnant, consult your doctor before trying the therapy. If you choose to do the therapy, let the reflexologist know you are pregnant.

- If you have a pacemaker, kidney stones or gallstones, let the reflexologist know.

FINDING A PRACTITIONER

Get a referral from your physician, from a physical therapist, or other therapist that you trust. There are no state laws regulating the practice of reflexology but there are certification programs. For a referral to a certified practitioner, you can also contact the American Reflexology Certification Board, (303) 933-6921. www.arcb.net.

Reiki

Common uses:
To promote self-healing, pain relief and relaxation.

Reiki (pronounced ray-key) is the channeling of spiritual energy through the practitioner's hands into the person receiving treatment. The theory is that the gentle laying on of hands breaks up blocked energy, rebalancing one's energy to promote healing. The term "reiki" comes from the Japanese *rei*, which means universal, and *ki*, meaning energy. Tibetan monks may have begun the practice, and it was introduced into Japan in the early 1900s. The deep relaxation induced by the therapy may also trigger the release of painkilling endorphins.

SCIENTIFIC EVIDENCE

Most research on reiki consists of case reports and small studies. However, several studies do show its painkilling effects. Patients with different kinds of pain, including pain resulting from cancer, had significant pain reduction after reiki treatment. [Cancer Prev Control. 1997 Jun; 1 (2): 108-13.] In a more recent study, cancer patients had less pain and better quality of life but no less pain medication following reiki treatment. [J Pain Symptom Manage. 2003 Nov; 26 (5): 990-7.] In a study of healthy people, reiki resulted in greater relaxation, less anxiety and lower blood pressure. [J Adv Nurs. 2001 Feb;33(4):439-45.]

And when five patients with chronic illnesses including lupus and fibromyalgia received 11 reiki treatments over nine weeks, they experienced increased relaxation, less pain and increased mobility. [Brewitt, Vittetoe, Hartwell]

SAFETY CONCERNS

• It should not be used in place of conventional care.

FINDING A PRACTITIONER

There is no national or state licensing for reiki. Ask your doctor, a physical or massage therapist you trust to recommend someone. There are three levels of reiki training. Training for the third one, or for Reiki Master, takes a year and is available only to those who have practiced the other two levels for at least 15 months. You can also contact the following organizations for referrals to a practitioner.

• The Reiki Alliance
(208) 783-3535
www.reikialliance.com

• American Reiki Master Association
(904) 755-9638
www.atlantic.net

Relaxation Techniques

Common uses:

To release tension and stress; to cope with pain and negative emotions.

Muscle relaxation and breathing techniques can help you learn to recognize and then release tension. The techniques are easy to learn and you can practice them at home. Deep breathing techniques taught in yoga tai chi and qi gong classes focus on breathing slowly and deeply to turn off the fight-or-flight response, lower blood pressure, ease panic attacks and control pain. Progressive muscle relaxation involves tensing and relaxing various parts of your body, muscle by muscle, focusing on the difference between tension and relaxation. Another technique is called a body scan in which you focus on the feeling in different parts of your body, section by section.

SCIENTIFIC EVIDENCE

A good deal of evidence suggests these techniques are effective in easing pain, depression, and anxiety. In a review of 25 studies, psychological therapies including relaxation techniques appeared to be more effective for those who have had rheumatoid arthritis only a short time that those in whom the condition is long-standing. [Arthritis Rheum. 2002 Jun 15; 476(3): 291-302.] Sixty-eight patients with rheumatoid arthritis had more mobility and were able to function more easily after muscle relaxation training for ten weeks. The improvements lasted up to 12 months. [Scand J Rheumatol. 1999; 28 (1): 47-53.] However, review of nine studies using relaxation techniques to address chronic pain deemed the studies inconclusive and poorly done. [J Adv Nurs. 1998 Mar; 27 (3): 476-87.]

SAFETY CONCERNS

- Tensing muscles may bring on cramps or pain at first. If you have rheumatoid arthritis or fibromyalgia and are experiencing a flare, start progressive muscle relaxation slowly. Tighten your muscles just enough to be aware of it and then release.

- Breathing exercises may make you lightheaded at first. Get up slowly after these or any relaxation exercise, checking your balance.

FINDING A PRACTITIONER

Ask your doctor to refer you to a physical or massage therapist or mental health practitioner who uses these techniques. Or check your local hospital and health organizations for stress reduction classes. You can also learn these techniques from audiotapes, videos and books.

Rolfing

Common uses:
To reduce stress, ease mobility, and reduce musculoskeletal and back pain.

Rolfing is a form of deep-tissue bodywork created by biochemist Ida P. Rolf in the 1930s. She wanted her therapy to address the way body structure affected function. It's based on the theory that physical and emotional stress can throw the body out of alignment, causing muscles and connective tissue (fascia) to become inflexible. Rolfing uses strong pressure from the knuckles, knees, elbows or fingers to stretch tightened fascia back into shape and to make them more flexible.

SCIENTIFIC EVIDENCE

Although there are few formal studies about rolfing, massage therapy in general has been found effective in promoting relaxation and improving pain. In a review of manipulation techniques for rheumatic diseases, researchers concluded that they are useful as a way to break the pain cycle – particularly for back and neck pain – and increase tolerance of exercise. But massage appears no more effective than other techniques such as physical therapy. [Med Clin North Am. 2002 Jan; 86 (1): 91-103.]

SAFETY CONCERNS

- Do not use this technique if you have rheumatoid arthritis or other inflammatory conditions.

- If you are pregnant, work only with an experienced practitioner and be sure to tell him you are expecting.

FINDING A PRACTITIONER

Ask your doctor, physical or massage therapist to recommend someone. You can also contact The Rolf Institute of Structural Integration at (800) 530–8875 or on www.rolf.org.

Rosen Method

Common uses:

To release muscle tension, increase flexibility, to enhance physical and emotional awareness.

The Rosen Method uses gentle touch to release muscle tension and to increase both inner and outer body awareness and experience. The originator of the method, Marion Rosen, developed the method through 50 years of work as a physical therapist and health educator. She noted that chronic muscle tension affects emotional health, and as tension is released, the patient can then explore the effect of and reasons for such chronic pain and tension. With the therapist's help, a patient can use his insights to break free of old patterns and become more receptive to new choices. Rosen began teaching her method in 1972 and now has 13 training centers.

SCIENTIFIC EVIDENCE

There have been no studies on the benefits of the Rosen Method although Rosen has been recognized by the International Somatics Congress for her contribution to the somatics field.

SAFETY CONCERNS

- The method can be a powerful experience, evoking emotions and memories. Check with your doctor before committing to the treatment, especially if you are receiving treatment for any psychological or medical condition.

FINDING A PRACTITIONER

Ask your doctor, physical therapist or a massage therapist you trust for a referral. You can also find practitioners through the Rosen Method Professional Association, (800) 893–2622 or www.rosenmethod.org. Certification takes two years of instruction followed by an internship lasting nine to 18 months. Many Rosen practitioners are also massage therapists. Talk to the practitioner before you commit to working with her, asking about her experience and background.

SAM or SAMe (S-adenosylmethionine)

Common uses:

To ease depression, treat fibromyalgia, osteoarthritis, migraine headaches.

SAM (S-adenosylmethionine) is a natural compound in the body, produced from methionine, a sulfur-contaning amino acid, and from adenosine triphosphate (ATP), an energy-producing compound. SAM helps form neurotransmitters, including serotonin and dopamine (which help boost mood), and helps maintain levels of glutathione, an antioxidant that helps protects cells from damage.

SCIENTIFIC EVIDENCE

A number of studies suggest that SAM is as effective as tricyclic antidepressants in addressing mild to moderate depression, and that it works faster (often within a week) and with fewer side effects. In December 2003, the Agency for Healthcare Research and Quality (AHRQ) reviewed 39 clinical trials and found SAM as effective as medication in treating patients for major depression. And a study at Massachusetts General Hospital found that SAM, taken simultaneously with antidepressants, was significantly more effective in relieving depression than the antidepressants alone. [American Psychiatric Association Annual Meeting, 2004] Studies regarding SAM and fibromyalgia have been mixed. A double-blind, placebo-controlled study found that SAM had no effect on those with fibromyalgia. [Scand J Rheumatol. 1997;26(3):206-11.] But in a more recent review of 16 randomized, placebo-controlled trials involving several antidepressants including SAM, reviewers concluded that fibromyalgia patients felt overall improvement. [J Gen Intern Med. 2000 Sep; 15 (9): 659-66.] Osteoarthritis studies have been more consistently positive. A double blind cross-over trial, for example, found that SAM was as effective as celecoxib (*Celebrex*) in managing symptoms of knee osteoarthritis, but some may dispute these findings. [BMC Musculoskelet Disord. 2004 Feb 26;5(1):6.] SAM can be expensive.

SIDE EFFECTS AND INTERACTIONS

- Large doses may cause upset stomach, nausea or insomnia.

- People with bipolar disorder should not take SAM; its antidepressant effects may cause mania.

- If you take antidepressants or anti-anxiety drugs, SAM may increase side effects. Talk to your doctor before taking.

SAFETY CONCERNS

- Do not treat severe depression with SAM.

- Theoretically, SAM may raise levels of homocysteine, a body substance associated with heart disease and stroke. However, a recent study at Massachusetts General Hospital found that SAM reduced homocysteine. It may be wise to ask your doctor to take a baseline homocysteine reading and monitor its levels while taking SAM.

DOSAGE

200 to 400 mg twice a day. Buy enteric-coated pills and take on an empty stomach. To avoid insomnia, take early in the day. SAM won't work without folic acid and B12 so make sure you have enough of these nutrients or take a supplement that includes them.

Sea Cucumber

Common uses:

To fight infection; to improve muscle strength; to treat arthritis, inflammation, muscle pain and high blood pressure.

Sea cucumber is a marine animal in the same family as starfish and sea urchins. Its sausage shape has earned it the cucumber moniker. In Asia people consider sea cucumbers a gourmet delicacy. But they have also been used for thousands of years as a medicine to help the body fight infection. They are also used to increase muscle strength, and to treat arthritis, inflammation, muscle pain and high blood pressure.

SCIENTIFIC EVIDENCE

Researchers believe that sea cucumbers improve the balance of prostaglandins, which control inflammation. They also contain substances such as chondroitins that help strengthen connective tissue and rebuild joint cartilage. However, there are no studies supporting sea cucumber's effectiveness in relieving arthritis.

SIDE EFFECTS AND INTERACTIONS

- At high doses, it may act as an anticoagulant.

SAFETY CONCERNS

- If you are pregnant or breastfeeding, taking any prescription or non-prescription medicine or supplements, or have any medical problems, especially heart or blood vessel disease, consult your doctor before taking.

- Stop taking if you have trouble breathing, hives, itchy skin or rash. You may be allergic to the medicine.

DOSAGE

Follow the dosage information on the bottle or consult with your doctor. Typical dosages are 500-2,000 mg per day, divided into morning and evening doses.

Selenium

Common uses:

To protect cells from oxidation damage; to boost the immune system.

Selenium is an essential mineral low in people with rheumatoid arthritis and other inflammatory conditions. Only a tiny amount is necessary to help protect cells from oxidation damage and boost the immune system, yet it exists in nearly every cell in the body. Its protective activity may help prevent cancer, cataracts and macular degeneration; protect against heart attack and stroke; help heal cold sores and shingles; and fight inflammation associated with lupus.

The best food source is a Brazil nut, but it's also plen-

tiful in seafood, poultry, meat and grains, especially oats
and brown rice.

SCIENTIFIC EVIDENCE

Studies indicate that those with rheumatoid arthritis have
lower levels of selenium in their blood than normal. [Biol
Trace Elem Res 1996; 53: 51-6.] And several studies suggest
that selenium may help relieve arthritis symptoms by con-
trolling the levels of destructive free radicals. [Analyst 1998;
123: 3-6.] But more studies are necessary to indicate whether
those with arthritis should take selenium supplements.

In one such study, 70 people with rheumatoid arthritis
who took selenium had a reduction in tender joints,
swelling, and early morning stiffness. But they were also
taking fish oil supplements.

SIDE EFFECTS AND INTERACTIONS

- May be most effective when taken in combination with
  400 IU of vitamin E.

SAFETY CONCERNS

- Take only in tiny doses. It can be harmful in large doses,
  and it is already in many multivitamins.

DOSAGE

50 to 200 mcg per day. The RDA is 55 mcg for women
and 70 mcg for men. Doses of 900 mcg have been toxic.
Most people get enough through diet alone. Symptoms of a
deficiency include muscle weakness and fatigue.

Serrapeptase

Common uses:

To treat inflammation and respiratory conditions; to help prevent plaque build-up in arteries

Serrapeptase is an enzyme produced in the intestines of silk worms. Studies suggest it reduces both inflammation and pain, and physicians in Europe and Asia often use it in place of NSAIDs. It has also successfully treated cystic breast disease and sinusitis.

SCIENTIFIC EVIDENCE

Serrapeptase appears to be a natural anti-inflammatory, reducing inflammation in a number of tissues. There are no studies yet documenting serrapeptase's effectiveness for arthritis or for cardiovascular health. Research is more definitive regarding its role in cystic breast disease and sinusitis. In a double-blind study, 70 patients with fibrocystic disease found serrapeptase reduced breast pain, swelling and firmness compared to placebo. [Singapore Med J. 1989; 30 (1): 48-54.] In a multicenter, double-blind, randomized trial, 193 subjects with ear, nose or throat inflammation had a significant reduction in symptoms, including pain, after three to four days of treatment with serrapeptase. [J Int Med Res. 1990 Sep-Oct;18(5):379-88.] In a study of 66 patients, those who took serrapeptase following surgery had a 50 percent decrease in swelling by day three. The control groups had none. [Fortschr Med. 1989 Feb 10;107(4):67-8, 71-2.]

SIDE EFFECTS AND INTERACTIONS

None

SAFETY CONCERNS

None

DOSAGE

Follow dosage instructions on the bottle or check with your doctor. Take enteric tablets or the enzyme will be killed by acid in the stomach.

Shark Cartilage

Common uses:

To promote bone and cartilage health; to treat the pain and inflammation of arthritis; to treat cancer.

Shark cartilage is a rich source of chondroitin and glycosaminoglycans (glucosamine-like compounds), natural substances thought to contribute to bone and cartilage strength and repair and which act as anti-inflammatories. Shark cartilage is also rich in calcium. The cartilage has gotten the most attention for its ability to slow the growth of blood vessels that nourish tumors.

SCIENTIFIC EVIDENCE

Although there is evidence that both chondroitin and glucosamine support bone and cartilage health, there are few studies about shark cartilage and arthritis. In general, chondroitin supplements derived from shark cartilage are not recommended because the cartilage may contain metals. Shark cartilage has received the most attention as a possible treatment for cancer. Some animal and in vitro studies suggest that shark cartilage slows the formation of blood vessels in tumors, stopping their growth. But patient outcome hasn't been good in clinical trials, and researchers are unsure how well the body even absorbs shark cartilage. [Biol Pharm Bull. 2001 Oct; 24 (10): 1097-101.]

SAFETY CONCERNS

• Shark cartilage may contain toxic metals.

DOSAGE

Shark cartilage supplements are not recommended because of metal content.

Shiatsu

Common uses:
To ease muscle tension, aches and pains.

Shiatsu (meaning "finger pressure") is a Japanese form of massage therapy much like acupressure. (See acupressure, p. 39). Practitioners use their fingers, thumbs, palms, elbows, knees and feet to apply pressure along the body's energy channels called meridians. The goal is to release blocked energy associated with illness. The scientific explanation is that shiatsu releases pain-killing endorphins and lowers stress hormones.

SCIENTIFIC EVIDENCE

Although there have been positive case studies, few clinical studies have been done on shiatsu. However, there have been positive studies about acupressure, shiatsu's therapeutic cousin, indicating that it can be effective at reducing pain.

SAFETY CONCERNS

- Avoid if you have an open wound, a rash or an infectious skin disease.

- Do not have if you are prone to blood clots, if you have recently had surgery or chemotherapy; if you have phlebitis or any circulatory ailment.

- Also avoid if you have a fracture or sprain.

FINDING A PRACTITIONER

Ask your physician or physical therapist to refer you to a practitioner, or contact the American Organization for Bodywork Therapies of Asia, (856) 782–1616 or www.aobta.org

Spray and Stretch

Common uses:
To reduce tension and offer pain relief.

Another massage technique, spray and stretch involves spraying a coolant such as flouri-methane over a painful area to cool the blood vessels and inactivate the tender points. The therapist then gently stretches the muscles in that area. Afterwards the muscles should feel looser, and the patient should have greater range of motion. The technique is most often used by a physician or physical therapist.

SCIENTIFIC EVIDENCE

There are no studies to confirm this method's effectiveness, although therapists recommend it and patients report relief. And massage in general has been found effective in relieving tension and pain.

SAFETY CONCERNS

- A practitioner should never press on an open wound, swollen or inflamed skin, bruises, surgical scars, varicose veins, broken bones, lymph nodes or tumors.
- Tell your practitioner if you are pregnant.

FINDING A PRACTITIONER

Ask your doctor or physical therapist to refer you.

St. John's Wort

Common uses:
To treat anxiety, insomnia, fibromyalgia.

St. John's wort is known as the "natural Prozac." It comes from a flowering plant that grows all over the world. Scientists aren't clear how St. John's wort works, but it may raise levels of serotonin, the neurotransmitter associated with mood and pain.

SCIENTIFIC EVIDENCE

A JAMA study on St. John's wort raised a stir in 2002 when it indicated that the herb was no better than placebo in relieving major depression. However, the study showed the same thing about sertraline hydrochloride (*Zoloft*), a selective serotonin reuptake inhibitor (SSRI). And 35 percent of studies of approved antidepressants also show those antidepressants no more effective than placebo. [Jama, 2002; 287: 1807]. A more recent meta-analysis of 30 studies using St. John's wort found the supplement as effective a synthetic antidepressants, and in mild to moderate depression, more effective with few side effects. [Fortschr Neurol Psychiatr. 2004 Jun;72(6):330-43.]

SIDE EFFECTS AND INTERACTIONS

- It may cause constipation, upset stomach, sedation, restlessness, dry mouth.

- It may also affect the way protease inhibitors, tricyclic antidepressants, cholesterol-lowering drugs, digoxin and theophylline are broken down by the liver, decreasing the levels of those drugs in the blood. And it may increase levels of SSRIs and MAO inhibitors, and up the side effects of antidepressants or anti-anxiety drugs. Talk to your doctor before taking.

- St. John's wort may cause increased sensitivity to sunlight when taken with other drugs that have the same effect such as tetracycline and tretinoin.

- St. John's wort may interfere with the effectiveness of birth control pills, causing bleeding and unwanted pregnancies.

SAFETY CONCERNS

- Do not treat severe depression with St. John's wort; it should be treated by a medical doctor.

- Do not take if you are pregnant or breast-feeding.

DOSAGE

300 mg a day (30 percent hypericin, the active ingredient in St. John's wort), three times a day. Take with meals to avoid upset stomach.

Stinging Nettle

Common uses:
To ease swelling and pain in sore joints.

Stinging nettle has been used for hundreds of years, particularly to treat arthritis. Herbalists believe that stinging yourself with the tiny stingers on a nettle plant injects chemicals that may cause an anti-inflammatory reaction. Until

2000, only folklore backed the claim. But that year, a British study found that nettles did lower pain in patients with osteoarthritis. There's more evidence, however, that ingested nettles inhibit the chemicals causing inflammation. The nettles contain boron, histamines and formic acid, all of which may help relieve pain. (See Boron, p. 60.)

SCIENTIFIC EVIDENCE

Some animal, in-vitro studies, and a few human studies indicate that stinging nettle has anti-inflammatory properties. A randomized controlled trial showed that after one week's treatment with nettle sting, patients with osteoarthritic pain in their thumbs or index fingers had significant reductions in pain and disability compared to the placebo group. [J R Soc Med. 2000 Jun;93(6):305-9.] And in an open, randomized German study, patients with osteoarthritis who took stinging nettle plus one fourth of their usual dose of NSAIDs did just as well as those taking the full dose of NSAIDs. [Chrubasik, 1997]

SIDE EFFECTS AND INTERACTIONS

- Skin redness and irritation may occur if you apply nettle topically.
- May cause upset stomach, fluid retention and hives.

SAFETY CONCERNS

- May cause an allergic reaction.
- Don't take nettle if you are pregnant or nursing.

DOSAGE

Capsules: as directed on the package. Tea: pour two-thirds cup boiling water over three to four teaspoons of dried leaves and steep for three to five minutes. Drink three to four times a day. Extract of leaves: two to five ml three times a day. Creams: As directed.

Sulfur (See also DMSO and MSM, pp. 105, 169)

Common uses:

To address the pain of arthritis; to address skin disorders and cystitis.

Sulfur is a mineral found primarily near hot springs and volcanoes. Its distinctive rotten-egg smell comes from its sulfur dioxide gas escaping into the air. In comes in two supplement forms – dimethyl sulfoxide (DMSO) and methylsulfonylmethane (MSM), both thought effective for pain. Sulfur is part of the chemical structure that builds protein and plays a role in producing collagen, a protein that keeps skin healthy. It also stokes metabolic processes and communication between nerve cells. Sulfur-containing mud baths (See balneotherapy, p. tk) are one of the oldest treatments for arthritis.

Good sources of sulfur include garlic, onions, brussels sprouts, asparagus, kale and wheat germ.

SCIENTIFIC EVIDENCE

In a study of those with osteoarthritis, researchers found that three weeks of sulfur baths reduced oxidative stress (the harm free radicals cause) and improved cholesterol levels more than those in the control group. [Forsch Komplementarmed Klass Naturheilkd. 2002 Aug; 9 (4): 216-20.] A review found sulfur a promising and safe treatment for a number of ailments including arthritis but also noted that human clinical trials are needed. [Altern Med Rev. 2002 Feb; 7 (1): 22-44.] A double-blind study of the effect of MSM on those with degenerative arthritis found an 82 percent improvement in pain at the end of six weeks compared to an 18 percent improvement in the control group. [Ronald M. Lawrence, UCLA School of Medicine, 2001]. In a German double-blind study, 112 patients with osteoarthritis of the knee, DMSO applied over three weeks was an effective pain reliever compared to placebo. [Fortschr Med. 1995 Nov 10; 113 (31): 446-50.] In a Swedish double-blind study of 150 patients with some kind of tendon-related pain, 44 percent of the patients were pain-free after 14 days of DMSO topical treatment compared to only 9 percent of the placebo group. [Fortschr Med. 1994 Apr 10; 112 (10): 142-6.] In an Irish study of 23 patients treated for interstitial cystitis with DMSO, 17 responded well to treatment. [Cathy McLean, Dept. of Urology, Gartnavel General Hospital, Glasgow, Scotland, 2000].

SIDE EFFECTS AND INTERACTIONS

- May cause stomach upset or even seizures.

- May cause headache or rash.

SAFETY CONCERNS

- Some people are allergic to sulfur so check with your doctor before using.

- Do not use if you are pregnant.

DOSAGE

There is no RDA for sulfur because a sufficient amount comes from a good diet. For arthritis, the recommended dose is 500 mg two times a day taken with meals to avoid an upset stomach. Used topically, apply doses of 60 to 90 percent DMSO one to three times a day.

Swedish Massage

Common uses:
To relieve muscle tension and promote relaxation.

Swedish, or European, massage is the method most Westerners are familiar with. It's a full-body treatment that involves kneading the top layers of muscles with oils. It's a particularly good introduction to massage for those with arthritis because it can be so gentle and relaxing.

SCIENTIFIC EVIDENCE

The results of formal studies are equivocal, despite lots of anecdotal evidence that massage is helpful, at least in the short term. A 2002 review of studies founds that massage is particular helpful for back and neck pain when compared to placebo but not any more effective than physical therapy or exercise. [Med Clin North Am. 2002 Jan; 86 (1): 91-103.] A British review was more lukewarm, noting that results were promising but the evidence was not clear that massage could control pain. [Clin J Pain. 2004 Jan-Feb; 20 (1): 8-12.]

SAFETY CONCERNS

- Massage can worsen high blood pressure, osteoporosis or circulation problems. Ask your doctors before trying.

- Do not have a massage if you are having a flare or are feeling ill. Do not massage areas where skin is broken, sore or painful.

- Tell the therapist if you are pregnant.

FINDING A PRACTITIONER

Ask your physician to refer you to a therapist. Or you can contact one of the following institutions:

- The National Certification Board for Therapeutic Massage and Bodywork
  (800) 296-0664
  www.ncbtmb.com

- The American Massage Therapy Association
  (847) 864-0123
  www.amtamassage.org

T-z

Tai Chi (Tai chi chuan)

Common uses:
Increasing flexibility; easing pain, stiffness and anxiety

Tai chi, also called tai chi chuan, is a form of Chinese martial arts practiced since the 1200s. It's designed to balance and enhance life energy or qi (pronounced chee). A principle of Chinese medicine is that ill health is caused by blocked or out-of-balance qi. By restoring balance, a person's body can begin to heal itself and resume normal functioning. Tai chi is based on a series of slow movements combined with deep breathing and mental focus. The gentle quality of the movements makes it an appealing exercise for those with arthritis, improving muscle strength without stressing joints.

SCIENTIFIC EVIDENCE

The growing data about tai chi is positive. In a 2004 review of four trials involving 206 participants, researchers found that tai chi had no ill effects on those with rheumatoid arthritis and significantly improved range of motion, particularly in the ankles. [Cochrane Database Syst Rev. 2004;(3):CD004849.] Yet another review of nine randomized controlled trials, 23 nonrandomized controlled studies, and 15 observational studies found tai chi benefits those with a range of chronic conditions including arthritis. Benefits included improvements in balance and strength, and flexibility. [Arch Intern Med. 2004 Mar 8;164(5):493-

501. Review.] A randomized, controlled clinical trial found that the symptoms in older women with osteoarthritis improved after 12 weeks of tai chi, as did their balance and function. [J Rheumatol. 2003 Sep;30(9):2039-44.] Another study found tai chi to be safe for those with rheumatoid arthritis. It may also help stimulate bone growth and strengthen connective tissue. [Am J Phys Med Rehabil. 1991 Jun; 70(3): 136-41.] In a later study at the University of Maryland combining qi gong (a form of exercise similar to tai chi) with mindfulness meditation, participants with fibromyalgia found their pain lessened and their depression, coping skills and functioning improved, changes that lasted at least six months following the study. [Altern Ther Health Med. 1998 Mar; 4 (2): 67-70.]

SAFETY CONCERNS

- Tai chi is safe, but you should tell your instructor about any physical limitations before you begin.

- Do only what feels comfortable. Most practitioners believe the internal focus is more important than the physical exercise.

FINDING AN INSTRUCTOR

There is no licensing or training requirement to be a tai chi instructor. Ask your doctor or physical therapist for a referral. You can also check with community centers, health clubs or a traditional Chinese medicine center. The Qi Journal website also lists instructors; www.qi-journal.com.

Thunder God Vine

Common uses:
To treat autoimmune diseases and inflammation.

Thunder god vine is a vine-like plant used to treat autoimmune diseases in China. Although there have been only a few studies, some show that the vine interferes with the production of chemicals responsible for immune responses and inflammation. Another study showed it inhibited pain chemicals. The active ingredient comes from the plant's roots.

SCIENTIFIC EVIDENCE

Although there are few well-designed studies, a growing body of data suggests the vine's positive effects. In a small double-blind, placebo-controlled trial, thunder god vine was shown to relieve joint pain and inflammation in those with rheumatoid arthritis more effectively than placebo And it caused fewer and less severe effects than most RA drugs. [Arthritis Rheum. 2002 Jul;46(7):1735-43.] In a randomized double blind, placebo controlled trial, patients with rheumatoid arthritis showed a 58 percent improvement rate when thunder god vine was applied topically compared to a 20 percent improvement rate in the placebo group. [J Rheumatol. 2003 Mar;30(3):465-7.]

SIDE EFFECTS AND INTERACTIONS
- May cause dry mouth, loss of appetite, nausea, diarrhea and rash.

SAFETY CONCERNS

- The leaves and flowers are poisonous and can cause death. Take preparations made from the root only.

DOSAGE

No standard dose has been established.

Trager Approach

Common uses:

To relieve chronic neuromuscular ailments such as back and neck pain, and stress-related conditions such as headache.

The Trager approach is a combination of massage and movement therapy. Begun in the 1920s by Dr. Milton Trager, the approach involves two parts. In the first part, the practitioner gently rocks, shakes and stretches your body, loosening tight muscles and joints. In the second part, the practitioner teaches you simple movements designed to reduce tension and increase mobility. The theory behind the therapy is that pain and reduced range of motion are the result of accumulated tension. If a person can relieve that tension and relearn how to move more easily, his physical pain and mental tension will ease.

SCIENTIFIC EVIDENCE

Although case studies and self-reports have suggested the therapy's effectiveness, there are few formal studies, and none related directly to arthritis. However, an early study found that two weeks of treatment with the Trager approach increased chest mobility in patients with chronic lung disease. [Phys Ther. 1986 Feb;66(2):214-7.] In a more recent clinical trial, the Trager approach eased the shoulder pain of those with spinal cord injury. [Arch Phys Med Rehabil. 2001 Aug;82(8):1038-46.] And among headache sufferers, the Trager approach decreased the frequency of headaches and the need for medication. [Altern Ther Health Med. 2004 Sep-Oct;10(5):40-6.]

SIDE EFFECTS AND INTERACTIONS

- May experience muscle soreness the day following a session.

SAFETY CONCERNS

- Do not use this method if you are in the first trimester of pregnancy.

- If you have a history of blood clots or have had joint surgery within the last three months, do not practice the Trager approach.

- If you have rheumatoid arthritis, tell the practitioner about any inflamed joints.

- Deep relaxation may cause anxiety. If so, you may need to see a mental health care professional to treat anxiety related to physical symptoms.

FINDING A PRACTITIONER

Check with your physician or physical therapist for a referral. You can also contact The Trager Institute, the only international organization certifying practitioners in the method, at (250) 337-5556 or www.trager.com.

Trigger Point Therapy

(See Neuromuscular Massage, p. 176)

Turmeric

Common uses:
To treat arthritis, inflammation, clogged arteries, bruises, bursitis; to prevent cancer.

Turmeric is a root and food spice related to ginger. It has long been used in Indian Ayurvedic medicine to treat ills including inflammation, clogged arteries, and bursitis. And in Chinese medicine it's been used to treat arthritis. The active ingredient is curcumin, which, combined with other ingredients such as boswellia and zinc, inhibits prostaglandins and stimulates the production of cortisol, both actions which relieve inflammation. Turmeric is also rich in anti-oxidants, which fight cell damage.

SCIENTIFIC EVIDENCE

In a randomized, double-blind study of 90 people with osteoarthritis, half of those who took a combination of spices including turmeric had significant and sustained pain relief compared to only 20 percent of placebo. [American College of Rheumatology 1999 annual scientific meeting]. In a similar study two years earlier, rheumatoid arthritis patients also experienced less pain and stiffness and had increased function compared to placebo. They also had lowered amounts of rheumatoid factor and interleukins, both markers of disease activity. [American College of Rheumatology 1997 annual scientific meeting]. Paw inflammation dropped significantly in arthritic rats given a combination of capsaicin and curcumin. [Mol Cell Biochem. 1997 Apr;169(1-2):125-34.] In a more recent randomized, double-blind, placebo-controlled study of dogs with osteoarthritis, however, the results were less promising. Although the treated dogs fared a bit better overall, the difference between the two groups was not significant. [Vet Rec. 2003 Apr 12;152(15):457-60.]

SIDE EFFECTS AND INTERACTIONS

- Prolonged use at high doses can cause upset stomach and other gastrointestinal difficulties.

SAFETY CONCERNS

- Do not use if you are pregnant or breastfeeding.

- Avoid if you have gallstones or any gall bladder problem, bile duct blockage, a blood-clotting disorder, or a history of stomach ulcers.

DOSAGE

400 mg three times a day in capsules or tablets.

Valerian

Common uses:
Treating insomnia and anxiety.

The root of this pink flowering perennial has been used as a sedative for centuries. It contains compounds, including valepotriates and valeric acid, thought to bind to a neurotransmitter called gamma-aminobutyric acid (GABA) thus improving sleep. That resembles how other sedatives work but valerian is not addictive, and you don't wake up foggy-headed the next morning. Instead valerian appears to relax the mind and body so that you can sleep. Health officials in much of Europe have approved it as a sleep aid.

SCIENTIFIC EVIDENCE

Recent research on valerian has yielded mixed results. A 2004 double-blind, placebo-controlled study of 16 sleep-disturbed patients found that valerian had no significant effect compared with placebo. [Phytother Res. 2004 Oct;18(10):831-6.] A 2003 randomized, controlled clinical trial had similarly bleak findings. Valerian wasn't any better than placebo in promoting sleep among 24 patients with chronic insomnia. [Complement Ther Med. 2003 Dec;11(4):215-22.] Yet a randomized, controlled clinical trial involving 202 patients with chronic sleep difficulties found valerian improved sleep as well as the sedative oxazepam. [Eur J Med Res. 2002 Nov 25;7(11): 480-6.] A double-blind, randomized, controlled German study also found that valerian works as well as the sedative benzodiazepine (*Librium*) with no withdrawal. [Wien Med Wochenschr. 1998;148(13):291-8.]

SIDE EFFECTS AND INTERACTIONS

- There are few side effects when used at correct doses, although headache, decreased concentration, dizziness, low body temperature and upset stomach sometimes occur.

- May cause drowsiness. Do not combine with others sleep aids, barbiturates, narcotics, antidepressants, alcohol or St. John's wort without speaking to your doctor first.

SAFETY CONCERNS

- May impair performance such as driving ability. Do not drive or operate machinery after taking valerian.

- The effects of long-term use are unknown.

- Pregnant and nursing women should not take valerian.

DOSAGE

150 to 300 mg of powdered extract (standardized to 0.8 percent valeric acid) in pill form 30 minutes before bedtime. If that is not effective, you can increase the dose to 600 to 900 mg.

Visualization

See Guided Imagery, p. 130.

Vitamins

Common uses:
General health and wellness.

The body needs 13 vitamins to function – A, C, D, E, K, the B vitamins (thiamin, riboflavin, niacin, pantothenic acid, biotin, B6, B12, and folate). Although the best way to get these vitamins is through diet, many people fall short. Some vitamins are thought to be helpful to those with arthritis in doses greater than the Recommended Daily Allowance (RDA). But not all vitamins are safe in large amounts, and studies don't yet show that vitamins in amounts greater than the RDA are helpful to healthy people.

If you have arthritis, it's a good idea to take a multivitamin. On top of that, you should get plenty of antioxidants (vitamins C, E, and A, or beta carotene, selenium, and flavonoids), available primarily in fruits and vegetables.

Lutein, found in leafy greens, and betacyptoxanthine, found in yellow and orange vegetables, both have been associated with lower risks of osteoarthritis.

Vitamin A (Beta carotene)

Common Uses:
To protect cells from free radical damage, which in turn may help prevent heart disease, and some cancers; for growth and development of the body; to boost the immune system.

Beta carotene, converted to vitamin A in our bodies, is one of a number of carotenoids that color fruits and vegetables yellow, orange and red. Vitamin A is essential for body development. It also boosts the immune system, and as an antioxidant, protects the body from damaging free radicals. Some studies have linked low vitamin A to development of lupus. Other studies suggest it may lower the risk of osteoarthritis.

SCIENTIFIC EVIDENCE

The Framingham Osteoarthritis Cohort Study involving 640 participants found beta carotene slowed progression of knee osteoarthritis by as much as 70 percent. [Arthritis Rheum. 1996 Apr;39(4):648-56.] One study, however, found an inexplicable increased risk. [Jordan] A more recent ongoing study of 23,000 people found beta carotene associated with a lowered risk of rheumatoid arthritis. [European Prospective Investigation of Cancer, 2004] Because the studies on arthritis and also on heart disease and cancer have been mixed, especially when beta carotene is taken in supplement form, many nutritionists do not recommend supplements.

SIDE EFFECTS AND INTERACTIONS

- If you eat too much beta carotene, it's possible your palms and soles may turn orange. If so, see your doctor, although in most cases, the coloration is harmless and will fade.

- If you eat too little, you may get dry skin, night blindness or greater risk of infection.

SAFETY CONCERNS

- Do not use beta carotene if you are pregnant; it can cause birth defects.

- It is almost impossible to overdose as the body excretes what it doesn't need.

DOSAGE

2,500 IU of beta carotene supplements per day for women; 5,000 IU for men. RDA: 10,000 IU (including what you eat).

Vitamin B

Common Uses:

Relieve fatigue and depression; promote healthy skin, eyes, hair, other organs.

The B vitamins – thamin (B1), riboflavin (B2), niacin (B3), pyridoxine (B6), folic acid (B9), cyanocobalamin (B12), pantothenic acid (B5), and biotin – are involved in many body processes, including energy production, digestion, and the nervous system. Because they work together, they are often taken as a B-complex supplement.

Some studies suggest that people with fibromyalgia have low levels of B vitamins, and symptoms of B deficiencies resemble those of fibromyalgia – confusion, muscle fatigue, depression, sleeplessness, anxiety, numbness or tingling in the hands or feet.

Scientific Evidence

Research indicates that there is a vitamin B12 deficiency in those with chronic fatigue syndrome and with fibromyalgia. [Neurology. 1993 Dec;43(12):2645-7.][Scand J Rheumatol. 1997;26(4):301-7.] But in a randomized controlled trial, injections of B12 had no effect on the fatigue of those with chronic fatigue syndrome. [Arch Intern Med. 1989 Nov;149(11):2501-3.] In another randomized controlled trial, homocysteine levels – associated with inflammation and fatigue – fell in patients with rheumatoid arthritis given B vitamins. [Scand J Rheumatol.

2003;32(4):205-10.] And a recent study showed that people treated for depression responded better if they had a higher level of B12 in their blood. [BMC Psychiatry. 2003 Dec 02;3(1):17.]

SIDE EFFECTS AND INTERACTIONS

- Thiamin (B1): No significant side effects. Sulfites (food preservatives) and black tea may lessen its effectiveness. Some drugs, such as diuretics, can cause a deficiency. Magnesium is needed to activate thiamin.

- Riboflavin (B2): Also no significant side effects. It may interact with some chemotherapy drugs, birth control pills, antibiotics, and psychiatric drugs. Check with your doctor before using. Riboflavin requires B6 to be active.

- Niacin (B3): Niacin can be toxic in large doses. It may cause skin flushing, upset stomach, and liver damage. It may also increase the effects of cholesterol-lower drugs, causing muscle pain and kidney damage. It may affect blood sugar levels as well. And you should avoid niacin if you have low blood pressure, glaucoma, gout, liver disease or ulcers. Do not take time-release niacin, which appears to affect the liver more. In short, consult your doctor before taking niacin.

- Pantothenic acid (B5): It has no significant side effects. High doses may affect the absorption of biotin and cause diarrhea.

- Pyridoxine (B6). High or even moderate doses of B6 can cause nerve damage when taken for long periods. Do not take more than 50 mg a day. B6 may reduce the effectiveness of anticonvulsant drugs. Those taking levodopa (L-dopa) should not take B6 unless combined with carbidopa (*Sinemet*).

- Folic acid (B9) Large doses may cause seizures in those with epilepsy and are dangerous to those with hormone-related cancers. They can also cause gas, nausea and loss of appetite. A high intake of folic acid can mask a B12 deficiency and vice versa, so take these vitamins together.

- Cyancobalamin (B12): No significant side effects. High intakes of folic acid can mask B12 deficiency and vice version so take these vitamins together. B12 interacts with antibiotics, methyldopa (*Aldomet*), azidothymidine (*AZT*), birth control pills, cimetidine (*Tagamet*), metformin (*Glucophage*), famotidine (*Pepcid*) soprazole (*Prevacid*), omeprazole (*Prilosec*), and rantidine (*Zantac*). One thousand mcg per day is sometimes recommended for fibromyalgia as an injection or tablet.

- Biotin: No significant side effects. Very high doses may affect the amount of insulin a person with diabetes needs.

Vitamin C

Common Uses:

To boost the immune system; heal wounds, ease colds and other infections; relieve asthma, prevent cataracts and certain cancers.

Vitamin C helps produce collagen, an essential protein in connective tissues, cartilage and tendons. High doses of vitamin C are associated with lowered risk of osteoarthritis.

SCIENTIFIC EVIDENCE

In a study of rheumatoid arthritis patients placed on a Mediterranean-type diet high in anti-oxidants, researchers found that the higher the blood levels of vitamin C, the lower the disease activity. [Nutr J. 2003 Jul 30;2(1):5.] In a multicenter, double-blind, randomized, placebo-controlled trial, Danish researchers found that vitamin C (calcium ascorbate) significantly reduced pain in those with osteo-arthritis of the hips or knees compared to placebo. [Ugeskr Laeger. 2003 Jun 16;165(25):2563-6. Danish.] And when twelve women with fibromyalgia were given a 500 mg blend of ascorbigen and broccoli powder for one month, they reported less sensitivity to pain and an improved quality of life. [Altern Med Rev. 2000 Oct;5(5):455-62.] Most dramatic are the results of an ongoing European Prospective Investigation of Cancer. In the study of 23,000 people, 73 had inflammatory polyarthritis. Those who consumed less than 40 mg of vitamin C a day had four times the risk of the polyarthritis. [Annals of Rheumatic Diseases, 2004]

SIDE EFFECTS AND INTERACTIONS

- The body excretes what it doesn't use, so high amounts aren't toxic. But doses above 2,000 mg can cause mouth ulcers, diarrhea, gas and bloating.

- High doses may increase the body's absorption of aluminum from antacids such as *Maalox* or *Mylanta*. Take vitamin C at least two hours before taking an antacid.

- Vitamin C increases iron absorption and decreases the absorption of copper.

- At high doses, it may decrease the body's ability to excrete acetaminophen (*Tylenol*), which could allow dangerous amounts to build up in the blood.

- If taken with tetracycline, it may increase levels of the antibiotic.

SAFETY CONCERNS

- It's considered safe. The body can only use up to 1,000 mg. Doses greater than that aren't beneficial.

- Those on dialysis or with kidney stones, kidney disease or gout should avoid high doses. They could increase the formation of kidney stones.

- Those with hemochromatosis, a disease resulting from too much iron, should not take vitamin C.

DOSAGE

500 mg daily.

Vitamin D

Common uses:

To protect bones and joints; prevent osteoporosis; offset the bone-stealing effects of corticosteroid medications such as prednisone.

Vitamin D comes primarily from exposure to sunlight and is necessary for bone growth and repair. Vitamin D also comes from dairy products, oily fish, liver, and fortified margarine and breakfast cereals. As we age, we become less efficient at producing D from sunlight or absorbing it from food.

SCIENTIFIC EVIDENCE

Some studies show that the progression of osteoarthritis slows in those who take higher levels of vitamin D. In a recent study of 221 patients with knee osteoarthritis, 48 percent of those with low levels of vitamin D have more pain and disability than those who did not. [Kristin Baker, Boston University, 2004] In a study of participants in the Framingham Study, researchers found that risk for knee osteoarthritis increased in those with low levels of vitamin D. [Ann Intern Med. 1996 Sep 1;125(5):353-9.] And in a study of elderly white women, development of hip osteoarthritis was associated with low levels of vitamin D. [Arthritis & Rheum, Volume 42, Issue 5, Pages 854 - 860Published Online: 22 Mar 2001]

SAFETY CONCERNS

- Excess doses (1,000 IU or more) may cause constipation, headaches, nausea, high blood pressure, seizures, growth retardation, and calcium deposits in the heart, blood vessels and kidneys.

DOSAGE

400-800 IU per day.

Vitamin E

Common uses:
To prevent heart disease, cancer; slow down aging.

Vitamin E is an anti-oxidant containing eight compounds: tocopherols and tocotrienols in four forms, altpha, beta, delta and gamma. Although E has gotten the most attention for its heart-healthy attributes, it also appears to help those with arthritis combat pain and boost immunity.

SCIENTIFIC EVIDENCE

Although vitamin E has been much touted for its role in preventing heart disease, a recent review of a number of studies found no protective effect. [Arch Intern Med. 2004 Jul 26;164(14):1552-6.] The research results about vitamin E are mixed. In a two-year, double-blind randomized placebo controlled study, vitamin E did not benefit those with knee osteoarthritis. [J Rheumatol. 2002 Dec;29(12):2585-91.] In a case controlled study at the University of North Carolina, Chapel Hill, researchers found that vitamin E was associated with a 30 percent lower risk of knee osteoarthritis in Caucasians but not in African-Americans. [Am J Epidemiol. 2004 May 15;159(10):968-77.] But in another double-blind randomized study, patients with osteoarthritis given 400 mg of vitamin E had just as much pain relief, reduction in swelling, and increase in mobility as those treated with 50 mg of diclofenac, an anti-inflammatory. [Z Rheumatol. 1990 Nov-Dec;49(6):369-73.]

SIDE EFFECTS AND INTERACTIONS

- Considered safe, it may nonetheless cause nausea, gas, diarrhea, heart palpitations and increased bleeding.

- If you take anticoagulant drugs, talk to your doctor before taking E. It may increase their effects.

- Do not take E before surgery.

- It may affect the effectiveness of tricyclic antidepressants and antipsychotic drugs.

- If you are taking cholesterol-lowering drugs, they may reduce the anti-oxidant effects of E.

DOSAGE

400 IU twice a day.

Wild Yam

Common uses:

To relax muscles and reduce inflammation; to relieve menstrual cramps, endometriosis and digestive problems; to fight cancer.

Wild yam is a climbing vine, unrelated to yams or sweet potatoes. The root was used by Aztecs and Mayans as a pain reliever, and some present day herbalists believe it addresses everything from pain to menopausal symptoms. However, current evidence is scarce.

SCIENTIFIC EVIDENCE

The studies are few and have yielded mixed results. In an in vitro study, diosgenin, the active ingredient in wild yam, significantly inhibited inflammatory substances active in rheumatoid arthritis. [Int Immunopharmacol. 2004 Nov;4(12):1489-97.] In another study, diosgenin inhibited the growth of synoviocytes, the cells that promote inflammation and joint destruction in rheumatoid arthritis. [Arthritis Res Ther. 2004;6(4):R373-83. Epub 2004 Jun 17.] In a cell study, diosgenin also appeared to inhibit leukemia cells. [Cancer Chemother Pharmacol. 2005 Jan;55(1):79-90. Epub 2004 Sep 14.] In a randomized clinical controlled trial, wild yam had little effect on 23 women suffering from menopausal symptoms. [Climacteric. 2001 Jun;4(2):144-50.]

SIDE EFFECTS AND INTERACTIONS

None known.

SAFETY CONCERNS

• Pregnant women should avoid wild yam.

DOSAGE

As directed on package labeling.

Yoga

Common uses:

To improve flexibility and promote relaxation.

Yoga is an ancient practice that combines mental, physical and spiritual training. With its emphasis on breath control, meditation and exercise, it can help lower blood pressure, increase energy, and may even lift mild depression. It also improves flexibility, muscle strength, and balance, and relieves stress.

There are several kinds of yoga, including bhakti, which focuses on spirituality; hatha, a physical yoga common in the U.S. involving gentle stretches or even vigorous workouts. Each variation involves holding positions called asanas and using slow, rhythmic breathing techniques called pranayama. The positions are done while attending to one's breath and physical sensations.

Yoga is an excellent exercise for those with arthritis because of its focus on gentle stretching, meditation, and the ability to pace oneself. The best way to learn yoga is to take a class so that a certified instructor can correct your postures.

SCIENTIFIC EVIDENCE

A number of studies over the past 12 years have indicated that yoga can improve strength and flexibility, and help control blood pressure, respiration and heart rate. [J Altern Complement Med. 2002 Dec;8(6):797-812.] A clinical randomized controlled trial found those with osteoarthritis in their hands had less pain and more flexibility after eight weeks of yoga.[J Rheumatol. 1994 Dec;21(12):2341-3.] In a randomized, single-blind controlled study of those with carpal tunnel syndrome, half the participants practiced yoga and half wore splints. After eight weeks, the yoga group had significant improvement in pain and grip strength.[JAMA. 1998 Nov 11;280(18):1601-3.] And in a clinical randomized controlled trial, depressed young adults reported significant decreases in depression, fatigue and anxiety after five weeks of yoga classes

SAFETY CONCERNS

- Done correctly, yoga is safe. However, be sure to tell your instructor about any physical limitations.

- Ask your doctors if there are poses you should avoid.

FINDING A PRACTITIONER

There are no licensing requirements for yoga instructors. But there are schools that offer certification. Ask your doctor or physical therapist for a referral. Or check with your local health clubs. Although the American Yoga Association does not offer referrals, you can call (921) 927- 4977, or check the website, www.american yogaassociation.org, for information about various types of yoga.

Zinc Sulfate

Common uses:

To boost the immune system, relieve pain, treat illness.

Zinc is an essential mineral in every body cell, used in almost all enzyme reactions, and necessary for hormones to work. It is essential for the immune system, for healing wounds, and for healthy skin. Many Americans lack enough zinc, and that may be especially true of those with autoimmune diseases like fibromyalgia, lupus and rheumatoid arthritis. Some animal studies suggest that zinc may lower pain. Zinc lozenges are also used to treat colds and flu.

SCIENTIFIC EVIDENCE

In a study surveying more than 29,000 older women, those with greater intakes of zinc were less likely to develop rheumatoid arthritis. [American Journal of Epidemiology, Feb. 2003] In a much earlier clinical trial, patients with rheumatoid arthritis who took zinc for 12 weeks had less swelling and morning stiffness than the controls.[Lancet. 1976 Sep 11;2(7985):539-42.] But in a small clinical trial of those with chronic inflammation, zinc had no effect. [Am J Clin Nutr. 1993 May;57(5):690-4.] In a randomized, placebo-controlled study of 100 patients, zinc significantly reduced symptoms of the common cold compared to placebo. [Ann Intern Med. 1996 Jul 15;125(2):81-8.]

SIDE EFFECTS AND INTERACTIONS

- More than 200 mg a day may cause nausea, vomiting and diarrhea. One hundred mg per day may lower HDL, the good cholesterol, suppress the immune system, and cause anemia. Talk to your doctor before taking.

- Zinc may also interfere with antibiotics. If you are taking zinc, take two hours after any antibiotic.

- High doses of iron or calcium may decrease the amount of zinc absorbed by the body.

SAFETY CONCERNS

- Some research has suggested that excess zinc is associated with Alzheimer's but more research is needed.

DOSAGE

30 mg per day.

ARTHRITIS FOUNDATION RESOURCES

For more information about the Arthritis Foundation, call our toll-free number, (800) 568-4045, or visit our website, www.arthritis.org. We offer a wide variety of information to people with arthritis, chronic pain, and arthritis-related diseases. You can find the Arthritis Foundation chapter nearest you through the toll-free number or website.

The mission of the Arthritis Foundation is to improve lives through leadership in the prevention, control and cure of arthritis and related diseases.